GREAT FOOD
EXPRESS
QUICK & EASY

THE *Skinny* CURRY RECIPE BOOK

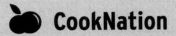

CookNation

THE SKINNY EXPRESS CURRY RECIPE BOOK
QUICK & EASY AUTHENTIC LOW FAT INDIAN DISHES UNDER 300, 400 & 500 CALORIES.

ISBN 978-1-909855-89-2

A CIP catalogue record of this book is available from the British Library

Photography: Kongsak/shutterstock

DISCLAIMER
Some recipes may contain nuts or traces of nuts. Those suffering from any allergies associated with nuts should avoid any recipes containing nuts or nut based oils.

This information is provided and sold with the knowledge that the publisher and author do not offer any legal or other professional advice. In the case of a need for any such expertise consult with the appropriate professional.

This book does not contain all information available on the subject, and other sources of recipes are available. This book has not been created to be specific to any individual's requirements.

Every effort has been made to make this book as accurate as possible. However, there may be typographical and or content errors. Therefore, this book should serve only as a general guide and not as the ultimate source of subject information.

This book contains information that might be dated and is intended only to educate and entertain.

The author and publisher shall have no liability or responsibility to any person or entity regarding any loss or damage incurred, or alleged to have incurred, directly or indirectly, by the information contained in this book.

www.cooknationbooks.com
www.bellmackenzie.com

CONTENTS

INTRODUCTION

Love Indian food but hate the calories?

Don't have time in the kitchen for over-complicated recipes with difficult to find and expensive ingredients?

The Skinny EXPRESS Curry Recipe Book is the jewel in the crown of curry lovers who want delicious, authentic, simple and inexpensive low calorie curries any night of the week.

We use delicate blends of spices to create mouth-watering Indian dishes from classic Indian specialties to popular favourites. We've stripped out lengthy prep times, uncommon spices and high fat, calorie heavy ingredients to create fresh and vibrant everyday healthy curries: all under 300, 400 and 500 calories each.

Our Skinny Express Curries are made for those craving a modern, healthier, lighter and quicker way of enjoying authentic Indian food with most dishes prepared and cooked in 30 minutes or less.

The recipes in this book are all low calorie Indian dishes serving 4, which makes it easier for you to monitor your overall daily calorie intake as well as those you are cooking for. The recommended daily calories are approximately 2000 for women and 2500 for men. Each skinny express recipe falls all under 300, 400 or 500 calories.

Many can be overwhelmed at the prospect of cooking Indian food in their own kitchen. The vast array of spices and often unfamiliar ingredients can look intimidating. Our express collection of skinny curries demystifies Indian cooking, taking away the fear and replacing it with confidence in your cooking. With just a handful of key spices you will easily create home cooked delicious Indian food in no time at all.

SKINNY EXPRESS CURRY TIPS

- For sauce based curries getting the correct consistency is key. If you feel like it's not thick enough, leave it to cook for a little longer with the lid off to thicken the sauce. Likewise if it's too thick, add some water or stock to loosen things up during cooking.
- Try to make sure your spices don't burn, this is really important. As we've really cut down on the oil to make the meals 'skinny' you might find adding a splash of water to the pan when you are cooking the dry spices helps.
- If you find any of your curries have a slight bitterness to them, add some sugar to counteract. Use small amounts of ½ tsp a time to make sure you don't over do it.
- Be confident. Feel free to use substitutes to suit your own taste and don't let a missing herb or spice stop you making a meal - you'll almost always be able to find something to replace it.

PORTION SIZES

The majority of recipes are for 4 servings. The calorie count is based on one serving. It is important to remember that if you are aiming to lose weight using any of our skinny express curry recipes, the size of the portion that you put on your plate will significantly affect your weight loss efforts. Filling your plate with over-sized portions will obviously increase your calorie intake and hamper your dieting efforts.
It is important with all meals that you use a correct sized portion, which is generally the size of your clenched fist. This applies to any side dishes of vegetables and carbs too.

SIDE DISHES

All the meals and sides in this book fall under 300, 400 & 500 calories.
You may choose to serve with a side dish depending on your diet or use one of these calorie counted side portions below.

Each side serves 4. The calories noted are PER SERVING.

- **300g/11oz mixed green salad: 20 calories**
- **200g/7oz long grain rice: 175 calories**
- **200g/7oz egg noodles 160 calories**

ALL RECIPES ARE A GUIDE ONLY

All the recipes in this book are a guide only. You may need to alter quantities and cooking times to suit your own appliances.

ABOUT COOKNATION

CookNation is the leading publisher of innovative and practical recipe books for the modern, health conscious cook.

CookNation titles bring together delicious, easy and practical recipes with their unique approach - easy and delicious, no-nonsense recipes - making cooking for diets and healthy eating fast, simple and fun.

With a range of #1 best-selling titles - from the innovative 'Skinny' calorie-counted series, to the 5:2 Diet Recipes collection - CookNation recipe books prove that 'Diet' can still mean 'Delicious'!

Turn to the end of this book to browse all CookNation's recipe books

CookNation

GREAT FOOD
EXPRESS
QUICK & EASY

Skinny
CURRY

CHICKEN DISHES

SERVES 4

SPICED CHICKEN & ONIONS

240 calories per serving (160)

Ingredients

- 500g/1lb 2oz chicken breast, cubed
- 1 tsp each turmeric & salt
- 1 tbsp vegetable oil
- 4 onions, peeled & sliced
- 3 garlic cloves, crushed
- 2 green chillies, deseeded & finely sliced
- ½ tsp each cumin & ginger
- 4 tbsp fat free Greek yogurt
- ½ tsp corn flour/starch
- 120ml/½ cup chicken stock
- 3 tbsp freshly chopped coriander/ cilantro

Method

1 Rub the chicken with the turmeric and salt.

2 Heat the oil in a large non-stick frying pan or wok and sauté the onions, garlic & chillies for a few minutes until the onions begin to soften.

3 Add the chicken to the pan and cook for 8-10 minutes or until the chicken is cooked through.

4 Meanwhile in a bowl whisk together the cumin, ginger, yogurt, corn flour and stock.

5 Stir this into the pan and cook for a couple of minutes or until the dish is piping hot and thick in texture.

6 Sprinkle with fresh coriander & serve.

CHEFS NOTE

Use some extra chillies in this dish if you want it super hot.

SERVES 4

PINEAPPLE & CHICKEN SKEWERS

200 calories per serving

Ingredients

- 1 tsp salt
- 2 tsp vegetable oil
- 1 garlic clove, crushed
- ½ tsp each chilli powder, coriander/ cilantro & cumin
- 2 tbsp fat free Greek yogurt
- 60ml/¼ cup pineapple juice
- 200g/7oz cherry tomatoes
- 400g/14oz chicken breast, cubed
- 2 red peppers, deseeded & cut into chunks
- 125g/4oz pineapple chunks
- 4 metal skewers

Method

1 Preheat the grill to a medium high heat.

2 In a bowl mix together the salt, oil, garlic, ground spices, yogurt & pineapple juice.

3 Add the whole cherry tomatoes, cubed chicken, pepper pieces & pineapple chunks and combine well.

4 Thread the chicken, tomatoes, peppers & pineapple chunks in turn onto the metal skewers.

5 Place the skewers under the grill and cook for 10-15 minutes or until everything is cooked through (turning occasionally).

CHEFS NOTE

If you have time: leave the chicken and vegetables to marinate in the yogurt for an hour or two. Don't worry if you don't, it will still taste great.

SERVES 4

BLACK PEPPER CHICKEN CURRY

255 calories per serving

175

Ingredients

- 2 tsp vegetable oil
- 2 onions, peeled & sliced
- 4 garlic cloves, crushed
- 2 green peppers, deseeded & sliced
- ½ tsp each fennel seeds, brown sugar, chilli powder, turmeric, ground ginger & ground black pepper
- 300g/11oz fresh tomatoes, chopped
- 2 tbsp tomato puree/paste
- 500g/1lb 2oz chicken breast, cut into strips
- 1 tsp garam masala
- 2 tbsp freshly chopped coriander/cilantro

Method

1 Heat the oil in a large non-stick frying pan or wok and sauté the onions, garlic, green peppers, fennel seeds & brown sugar for a few minutes until the onions begin to soften.

2 Add the chilli powder, turmeric, ginger, black pepper, tomatoes & puree and cook for 3-4 minutes keeping everything moving around the pan on a fairly high heat (add a splash of water if you find you need to).

3 Add the chicken to the pan, cover and whack up the heat for about 10 minutes or until the chicken is cooked through.

4 Stir through the garam masala, sprinkle with fresh coriander and serve.

CHEFS NOTE

Add a little chicken stock if you want more moisture in your curry.

SERVES 4

CASHEW CHICKEN CURRY

280
calories per serving

Ingredients

- ½ tsp cumin seeds
- 1 tsp coriander/cilantro seeds
- 3 tbsp cashew nuts
- 250ml/1 cup water
- 1 tsp vegetable oil
- 1 onion, peeled & sliced
- 4 garlic cloves, crushed
- ½ tsp turmeric
- 2 tsp freshly grated ginger
- 2 green chillies, deseeded & very finely sliced
- 500g/1lb 2oz chicken breast, cut into thick diagonal strips
- 2 tbsp freshly chopped coriander/cilantro

Method

1 Quickly cook the cumin & coriander seeds in a dry pan on a medium heat for about 60 seconds. When you begin to smell the aroma remove from the pan and smash with a pestle and mortar.

2 Place the cashew nuts and water into a blender and whizz to make a smooth paste (add a little more water if you need to).

3 Heat the oil in a large non-stick frying pan or wok and sauté the onions, garlic, turmeric, ginger, chillies & smashed seeds for a few minutes until the onions begin to soften.

4 Add the chicken to the frying pan along with the cashew paste and simmer for 10-12 minutes or until the chicken is cooked through (add a little water or chicken stock to the pan now and again if you need to).

5 Sprinkle with fresh coriander and serve.

CHEFS NOTE

Alter the consistency of the dish by adding more water or cooking for a little longer to thicken the sauce.

LACCHA CHICKEN STRIPS

SERVES 4

295 calories per serving

Ingredients

- 1 tsp vegetable oil
- 2 onions, peeled & sliced
- 3 garlic cloves, crushed
- 1 tsp freshly grated ginger
- 1 tsp each cumin seeds
- 1 green pepper, deseeded & very finely sliced
- 1 green chilli, deseeded & very finely sliced
- 500g/1lb 2oz chicken breast, cut into strips
- 1 tbsp ground almonds
- 1 tbsp desiccated coconut
- 4 tbsp fat free Greek yogurt
- 120ml/½ cup chicken stock
- 2 tbsp freshly chopped coriander/ cilantro

Method

1 Heat the oil in a large non-stick frying pan or wok and sauté the onions, garlic, ginger & cumin seeds for a few minutes until the onions begin to soften.

2 Add the peppers, chilli & chicken strips to the frying pan and stir-fry on a high heat for 3-4 minutes or until the chicken is sealed.

3 Stir through the ground almonds, coconut & yogurt and cook for 2 minutes. Add the chicken stock and simmer for a further 5 -8 minutes or until the chicken is cooked through and the sauce has thickened.

4 Sprinkle with fresh coriander and serve with salad, rice or Indian bread.

CHEFS NOTE

Reserve a little of the sliced pepper to use as a garnish if you wish.

SERVES 4

ROASTED CUMIN SEED CHICKEN

275 calories per serving

Ingredients

- 2 tsp cumin seeds
- 1 tsp coriander/cilantro seeds
- 1 tbsp vegetable oil
- 2 onions, peeled & sliced
- 2 garlic cloves, crushed
- 1 tsp freshly grated ginger
- ½ tsp cardamom seeds
- 2 green chillies, deseeded & very finely sliced
- 500g/1lb 2oz chicken breast, cut into thick diagonal strips
- 2 tbsp freshly chopped coriander/cilantro

Method

1 Quickly cook the cumin & coriander seeds in a dry pan on a medium heat for about 60 seconds. When you begin to smell the aroma remove from the pan and smash with a pestle and mortar.

2 Heat the oil in a large non-stick frying pan or wok and sauté the onions, garlic, ginger & cardamom seeds for a few minutes until the onions begin to soften.

3 Add the chicken and smashed seeds to the frying pan and stir-fry on a high heat for 10-12 minutes or until the chicken is cooked through (add a little water or chicken stock to the pan now and again if you need to).

4 Sprinkle with fresh coriander and serve with salad, rice or Indian bread.

CHEFS NOTE

Roasting the seeds will fill your kitchen with mouth-watering aromas but be careful not to burn the spices.

SERVES 4

KERALAM CHICKEN CURRY

300 calories per serving

220

Ingredients

- 2 tsp vegetable oil
- 2 onions, peeled & sliced
- 2 garlic cloves, crushed
- 1 tsp freshly grated ginger
- 4 curry leaves
- 1 tsp each fennel seeds & chilli powder
- 2 tsp ground coriander/cilantro
- ½ tsp turmeric & ground black pepper
- 500g/1lb 2oz chicken breast, cut into strips
- 200g/7oz cherry tomatoes, roughly chopped
- 200g/7oz green beans
- 120ml/½ cup low fat coconut milk
- 2 tbsp freshly chopped coriander/cilantro

Method

1 Heat the oil in a large non-stick frying pan or wok and sauté the onions, garlic & ginger for a few minutes until the onions begin to soften.

2 Add the curry leaves, fennel seeds & all the dry spices and cook for a further 5 minutes before adding the chicken and cooking for 3-4 minutes to seal the meat. While you are cooking keep everything moving around the pan on a fairly high heat (adding a splash of water every now and again if you need to).

3 Add the tomatoes, green beans & coconut milk and cook for 10 minutes or until the chicken is cooked through.

4 Sprinkle with fresh coriander and serve with rice, salad or warm bread.

CHEFS NOTE

The Kerelam area of Indian is famed for its coconut milk curries.

SERVES 4

MURGH DRUMSTICK CURRY

380 calories per serving

Ingredients

- 2 tsp vegetable oil
- 2 onions, peeled & sliced
- 1 red chilli, deseeded & finely chopped
- 4 garlic cloves, crushed
- ½ tsp each brown sugar, turmeric & ground ginger
- 125g/4oz fresh tomatoes, chopped
- 1 tbsp tomato puree/paste
- 8 skinless chicken drumsticks (each weighing 100g/3½oz)
- 2 tbsp fat free Greek yogurt
- 120ml/½ cup chicken stock (or water)
- 1 tsp garam masala
- 2 tbsp freshly chopped coriander/ cilantro

Method

1 Heat the oil in a large non-stick frying pan or wok and sauté the onions, chilli, garlic & brown sugar for a few minutes until the onions begin to soften.

2 Add the turmeric, ginger, tomatoes & puree and cook for 3-4 minutes keeping everything moving around the pan on a fairly high heat (add a splash of water if you find you need to).

3 Add the chicken to the pan. Stir through the yogurt, add the stock, cover and whack up the heat. Simmer for 15 minutes, stirring occasionally, or until the chicken is cooked through and the sauce thickens up.

4 Stir through the garam masala, sprinkle with fresh coriander and serve.

CHEFS NOTE

Murgh is the Indian cooking term for Chicken.

SERVES 4

PALAK CHICKEN CURRY

240 calories per serving

Ingredients

- 2 tsp vegetable oil
- 2 onions, peeled & sliced
- 4 garlic cloves, crushed
- 4 green cardamoms
- 1 tsp each fresh brown sugar, chilli powder, cumin & ground coriander/cilantro
- ½ tsp each ground cinnamon & turmeric
- 300g/11oz tomatoes, chopped
- 2 tbsp tomato puree/paste
- 500g/1lb 2oz chicken breast, cut into strips
- 200g/7oz spinach
- 2 tbsp lemon juice

Method

1 Heat the oil in a large non-stick frying pan or wok and sauté the onions, garlic, green cardamoms & brown sugar for a few minutes until the onions begin to soften.

2 Add the chilli powder, cumin, coriander, cinnamon, turmeric & tomatoes and cook for 3-4 minutes keeping everything moving around the pan on a fairly high heat (add a splash of water if you find you need to).

3 Add the chicken to the pan and whack up the heat: stir-frying for 8-10 minutes or until the chicken is cooked through. Quickly stir through the spinach and lemon juice for 30 seconds. Check the seasoning and serve with green vegetables or rice.

CHEFS NOTE

This dish is good with the spinach served crunchy but you can wilt it completely before serving if you prefer.

SERVES 4

REAL PAN FRIED CHICKEN JHALFREZI

275 calories per serving

195

Ingredients

- 500g/1lb 2oz chicken breast, cut into strips
- 1 tsp each turmeric & chilli powder
- 4 tbsp fat free Greek yogurt
- 1 tsp vegetable oil
- 2 onions, peeled & sliced
- 2 garlic cloves, crushed
- 1 tsp freshly grated ginger
- 3 green peppers, deseeded & sliced
- 200g/7oz ripe cherry tomatoes, quartered
- 2 tbsp lemon juice
- 200g/7oz spinach leaves
- 2 tbsp freshly chopped coriander/ cilantro

Method

1 Mix together the chicken strips, turmeric, chilli powder & yogurt and put to one side.

2 Meanwhile heat the oil in a large non-stick frying pan or wok and sauté the onions, garlic & ginger for a few minutes until the onions begin to soften.

3 Add the yogurt chicken strips to the frying pan and stir-fry on a high heat for 3-4 minutes or until the chicken is sealed.

4 Add the peppers & tomatoes and stir-fry for a further 5-7 minutes or until the chicken is cooked through and the peppers are tender.

5 Stir though the lemon juice and serve piled over a bed of spinach leaves with the coriander sprinkled over the top.

CHEFS NOTE

Jhalfrezi is a classic Indian stir-fry, which bears little resemblance to the version sold in most western restaurants.

Skinny CURRY

MEAT DISHES

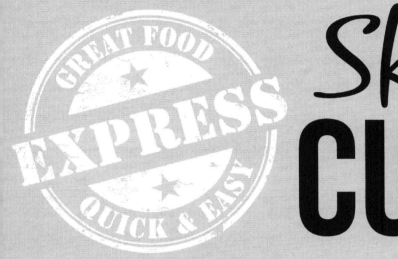

SERVES 4

LAMB KOFTA & HOT SAUCE

320 calories per serving

Ingredients

Kofta Ingredients:

- 500g/1lb 2oz lean, minced/ground lamb
- 2 garlic cloves
- 1 onion
- 1 tsp each cumin & chilli powder
- Small handful of fresh coriander/cilantro
- 1 egg

Sauce Ingredients:

- 4 tbsp fat free Greek yogurt
- 2 tbsp tomato puree/paste
- 1 garlic clove, crushed
- 1 tsp each chilli powder, salt, garam masala & cumin
- 1 tbsp vegetable oil
- 500ml/2 cups water

Method

1 First make the kofta: place all the kofta ingredients into a food processor and pulse until you have a fine mixture.

2 Remove the mixture from the food processor and, using your hands, shape into approx. 20 small balls. Put to one side while you make the sauce.

3 Combine all the sauce ingredients together, except the oil and water.

4 Heat the oil in a large non-stick frying pan or wok and add the sauce, gently cook for a minute or two.

5 Stir through the water and add the kofta balls. Cover and gently cook for 10-15 minutes, stirring occasionally, or until the koftas are cooked through and piping hot.

6 Serve with roti bread or salad.

CHEFS NOTE

Make sure the yogurt is at room temperature when you cook to avoid it splitting and spoiling.

SERVES 4

EASY BEEF KEEMA

475 calories per serving

Ingredients

- 1 tsp vegetable oil
- 2 onions, peeled & sliced
- 2 garlic cloves, crushed
- 400g/1lb 2oz lean, mince/ground beef
- 200g/7oz fresh tomatoes, roughly chopped
- 1 tsp each turmeric, coriander/cilantro & chilli powder
- 250g/9oz basmati rice
- 500ml/2 cups beef or chicken stock
- 200g/7oz mixed vegetables
- 2 tbsp freshly chopped coriander/ cilantro

Method

1. Heat the oil in a large non-stick frying pan or wok and sauté the onions & garlic for a few minutes until the onions begin to soften.
2. Add the beef and move around the pan to brown it off for a minute or two.
3. Add the tomatoes, turmeric, coriander & chilli powder and cook for 3 minutes. Meanwhile rinse the rice in cold water and add this to the pan along with the hot stock.
4. Cover and leave to cook for 10 minutes (adding more stock or water throughout cooking to make sure the rice is tender).
5. Add the vegetables and cook for 5 minutes longer, or until the rice is tender, the stock has been absorbed and the beef is cooked through.
6. Season and sprinkle with fresh coriander.

CHEFS NOTE

Try serving with a dollop of fat free yogurt.

SERVES 4

CORIANDER BEEF PATTIES

310 calories per serving

Ingredients

- 500g/1lb 2oz lean, minced/ground beef
- 5 garlic cloves
- 1 red onion
- ½ tsp ground ginger
- 1 tsp each cumin, chilli powder & salt
- Small handful of fresh coriander/cilantro
- 1 egg
- 125g/5oz fresh peas

Method

1 Preheat the grill to a medium high heat.

2 Place the beef, garlic cloves, onion, dried spices, salt, fresh coriander & egg into a food processor and whizz until you have a fine mixture.

3 Remove the mixture from the food processor and, using your hands, shape into 12 small patties.

4 Place the patties under the grill and, turning once, cook for 10-15 minutes or until everything is cooked through and piping hot.

CHEFS NOTE

Serve with pitta bread, raita and slices of raw red onion.

SERVES 4

GROUND LAMB SKEWERS

280 calories per serving

Ingredients

- 500g/1lb 2oz lean, minced/ground lamb
- 5 garlic cloves
- Small handful mint leaves
- 1 tsp each coriander/cilantro, chilli powder, garam masala & salt
- 1 egg
- 8 small metal skewers

Method

1 Preheat the grill to a medium high heat.

2 Place the lamb, garlic cloves, mint leaves, dried spices, salt & egg into a food processor and whizz until you have a fine mixture.

3 Remove this from the food processor and, using your hands, shape into 8 thick sausages around each skewer (so you end up with a 'sausage-on-a-stick').

4 Place the skewers under the grill and, turning occasionally, cook for 10-15 minutes or until everything is cooked through and piping hot.

5 Season and serve.

CHEFS NOTE

Serve with some cooling yoghurt and a large green salad.

LAMB & FRESH PEA PATTIES

SERVES 4

310 calories per serving

Ingredients

- 500g/1lb 2oz lean, minced/ground lamb
- 5 garlic cloves
- 1 onion
- 1 tsp each coriander/cilantro, chilli powder & salt
- ½ tsp ground ginger
- 1 egg
- 125g/5oz fresh peas

Method

1 Preheat the grill to a medium high heat.

2 Place the lamb, garlic cloves, onion, dried spices, salt & egg into a food processor and whizz until you have a fine mixture.

3 Remove the blade from the food processor and combine in the fresh peas.

4 Remove the mixture from the food processor and, using your hands, shape into 12 small patties.

5 Place the patties under the grill and, turning once, cook for 10-15 minutes or until everything is cooked through and piping hot.

6 Season and serve.

CHEFS NOTE

This is lovely served with a simple salad or a veggie side dish.

SERVES 4

MATAR KEEMA

350 calories per serving

Ingredients

- 1 tsp vegetable oil
- 2 onions, peeled & sliced
- 2 garlic cloves, crushed
- 1 tsp freshly grated ginger
- 4 green cardamoms
- ½ tsp each ground black pepper, salt & chilli powder
- 1 tsp each ground coriander/cilantro, cumin
- 4 tbsp tomato puree/paste
- 500g/1lb 2oz lean minced/ground beef
- 200g/7oz frozen peas
- 200g/7oz green beans, halved
- 2 green chillies, deseeded & finely chopped
- 120ml/½ cup beef stock or water
- 4 tbsp fat free Greek yogurt
- 2 tbsp freshly chopped coriander/cilantro

Method

1 Heat the oil in a large non-stick frying pan or wok and sauté the onions, garlic, ginger & cardamoms on a medium heat for a few minutes until the onions begin to soften.

2 Add the pepper, salt, chilli powder, ground coriander & cumin and move around the pan for 2-3 minutes (add a splash of water to the pan if you find the spices are sticking).

3 Stir through the tomato puree. Add the beef, peas, green beans & chopped chillies and cook for a further 5 minutes. Add the stock and cook for 10 minutes or until the beef is cooked through and the stock has been absorbed.

4 Stir though the Greek yoghurt, divide into bowls and sprinkle with fresh coriander.

CHEFS NOTE

Greek yogurt is best added to cooking when it is at room temperature as it discourages 'splitting'.

SERVES 4

SIRLOIN STEAK & GREEN BEAN CURRY

320 calories per serving

Ingredients

- 1 tbsp vegetable oil
- 2 onions, finely chopped
- 2 garlic cloves, crushed
- 2 celery stalks, chopped
- 2 green chillies, deseeded & finely sliced
- ½ tsp each ground turmeric, coriander/cilantro, cumin & salt
- 500g/1lb 2oz lean sirloin steak, thickly sliced
- 3 tbsp tomato puree/paste
- 200g/7oz green beans
- 120ml/½ cup beef stock/broth
- 3 tbsp freshly chopped basil

Method

1 Heat the oil in a large non-stick frying pan or wok and sauté the onions, garlic, celery, & chillies for a few minutes until the onions begin to soften.

2 Add the ground spices & salt and cook for a minute or two long (add a splash of water to the pan if you need to).

3 Add the steak slices and stir-fry on a high heat for 2 minutes. Stir in the puree, beans & stock. Cover and simmer for 2-3 minutes or until the steak is cooked to your liking and the beans are tender.

4 Sprinkle with fresh basil and serve with salad, rice or Indian bread.

CHEFS NOTE

Trim the steak of all visible fat before slicing.

SERVES 4

CREAMY PAPRIKA CURRY

285 calories per serving

Ingredients

- 2 tsp vegetable oil
- 1 onion, finely chopped
- 2 green peppers, deseeded & thinly sliced
- 3 garlic cloves, crushed
- ½ tsp each turmeric, chilli powder, coriander/cilantro, cumin, ginger & salt
- 2 tsp paprika
- 500g/1lb 2oz pork tenderloin, sliced into strips
- 2 tbsp tomato puree/paste
- 4 tbsp fat free Greek yogurt

Method

1 Heat the oil in a large non-stick frying pan or wok and sauté the onions, peppers & garlic for a few minutes until the onions begin to soften.

2 Add the ground spices & salt and cook for a minute or two long (add a splash of water to the pan if you need to loosen it up).

3 Add the pork slices and stir-fry on a high heat for 4-5 minutes. Stir in the puree & yoghurt. Cover and simmer for 2-3 minutes or until the pork is cooked through.

CHEFS NOTE

Try garnishing with some ground almonds and serve with lots of steamed vegetables.

GREAT FOOD EXPRESS QUICK & EASY

Skinny CURRY

SEAFOOD DISHES

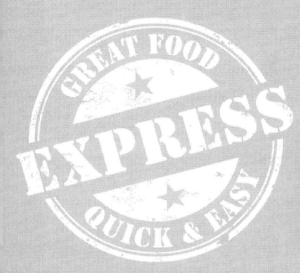

SERVES 4

GREEN CHILLI PRAWNS & RICE

380 calories per serving

Ingredients

- 1 tsp vegetable oil
- 2 onions, peeled & sliced
- 2 garlic cloves, crushed
- 200g/7oz fresh tomatoes, roughly chopped
- 1 tsp each turmeric & paprika
- 2 green chillies, deseeded & finely chopped
- 300g/11oz basmati rice
- 500ml/2 cups chicken or vegetable stock
- 500g/1lb 2oz king prawns, peeled
- 200g/7oz green beans
- 2 tbsp freshly chopped coriander/cilantro

Method

1 Heat the oil in a large non-stick frying pan or wok and sauté the onions & garlic for a few minutes until the onions begin to soften.

2 Add the tomatoes, turmeric & chillies and cook for 3 minutes. Meanwhile rinse the rice in cold water and add this to the pan along with the hot stock.

3 Cover and leave to cook for 10 minutes (adding more stock or water throughout cooking to make sure the rice is tender).

4 Add the prawns and green beans and cook for 5-7 minutes longer, or until the rice is tender, the stock has been absorbed and the prawns are cooked through.

5 Season and sprinkle with fresh coriander.

CHEFS NOTE

A tablespoon of coconut cream stirred in towards the end of cooking is nice too.

SERVES 4

TANDOORI PRAWN SKEWERS

160 calories per serving

Ingredients

- 4 garlic cloves, crushed
- 2 tsp freshly grated ginger
- 1 tsp each chilli powder, coriander/cilantro & cumin
- 2 tbsp fat free Greek yogurt
- ½ tsp salt
- 600g/1lb 5oz raw king prawns, shelled
- 4 metal skewers
- Lime wedges

Method

1 Preheat the grill to a medium high heat.

2 Mix the garlic, ginger, chilli powder, coriander, cumin, yogurt and salt together.

3 Smother the prawns in this mixture and thread the prawns in turn onto the skewers (if you have the time you could prepare this dish and leave to marinade overnight before cooking).

4 Place the skewers under the grill and cook for 4-5 minutes each side or until the prawns are cooked through.

5 Season and serve with lime wedges.

CHEFS NOTE

Serve with lots of green salad or a tomato and onion salad.

SERVES 4

GOAN FISH CURRY

250 calories per serving

Ingredients

- 500g/1lb 2oz boneless, meaty white fish fillets, cubed
- 1 tsp turmeric
- ½ tsp salt
- ½ tsp cumin seeds
- 2 tsp coriander/cilantro seeds
- 1 tbsp vegetable oil
- 1 onion, peeled & sliced
- 2 garlic cloves, crushed
- 1 tsp freshly grated ginger
- ½ tsp chilli powder
- 1 tsp tamarind paste
- 250ml/1 cup low fat coconut milk
- 400g/14oz tinned chopped tomatoes
- 2 tbsp freshly chopped coriander/cilantro

Method

1 First rub the cubed fish with a little salt & turmeric.

2 Quickly cook the cumin & coriander seeds in a dry non-stick frying pan or wok on a medium heat for about 60 seconds. When you begin to smell the aroma remove from the pan and smash with a pestle and mortar.

3 Heat the oil in the same pan and fry the fish pieces for 1 minute each side until sealed. Remove to a plate and add the onions, garlic, ginger & chilli powder to the frying pan. Sauté for a few minutes until the onions soften (add a splash of water to the pan now and again if you need to).

4 Add the tamarind paste, smashed seeds, coconut milk & chopped tomatoes and cook on a hard simmer for 5 minutes.

5 Add the fish pieces and gently cook for 4-8 minutes or until the fish is piping hot.

6 Sprinkle with fresh coriander and serve.

CHEFS NOTE

This simple fish curry is a staple meal for coastal Indian communities.

SERVES 4

CASHEW & COCONUT FISH CURRY

305 calories per serving

Ingredients

- 600g/1lb 5oz boneless, meaty white fish fillets, cubed
- 1 tsp turmeric
- ½ tsp salt
- ½ tsp cumin seeds
- 2 tsp coriander/cilantro seeds
- 1 tbsp cashew nuts
- 2 tbsp desiccated coconut
- 250ml/1 cup water
- 1 tbsp vegetable oil
- 1 onion, peeled & sliced
- 4 garlic cloves, crushed
- 2 tsp freshly grated ginger
- 2 green chillies, deseeded & very finely spiced
- 1 green pepper, deseeded & sliced
- 2 tbsp freshly chopped coriander/cilantro

Method

1 First rub the cubed fish with a little salt & turmeric.

2 Quickly cook the cumin & coriander seeds in a dry non-stick frying pan or wok on a medium heat for about 60 seconds. When you begin to smell the aroma remove from the pan and smash with a pestle and mortar.

3 Place the cashew nuts, desiccated coconut & water into a blender and whizz to make a smooth paste (add a little more water if you need to).

4 Heat the oil in the same pan and fry the fish pieces for 1 minute each side and remove to a plate. Add the onions, garlic, ginger, chillies, peppers & smashed seeds to the pan and sauté for a few minutes until the onions begin to soften.

5 Add the cashew & coconut paste to the pan and simmer for 5 minutes. Add the fish pieces and cook for a further 5-8 minutes or until the fish is piping hot.

6 Sprinkle with fresh coriander and serve.

CHEFS NOTE

Use any type of firm meaty white fish you prefer.

SERVES 4

TANDOORI FISH

210
calories per serving

Ingredients

- 4 large boneless white fish fillets (each weighing 175g/6oz)
- 2 tbsp lemon juice
- ½ tsp salt
- 6 garlic cloves
- Small bunch of fresh coriander/cilantro
- 1 tsp vegetable oil
- 1 tbsp water
- ½ tsp each chilli powder & ground ginger
- 1 tsp each paprika & mango powder

Method

1. Brush the fish with lemon juice & salt and set to one side
2. Preheat the grill to a medium high heat.
3. Place all the other ingredients in a food processor and pulse until finely chopped into a paste (add a little more water if you need to loosen it up).
4. Cover the fish fillets with the paste and grill for 8-12 minutes or until cooked through.
5. Season and serve.

CHEFS NOTE

Try serving with cool yogurt raita and salad or roti bread.

SERVES 4

FAST CREAMY KING PRAWNS

225 calories per serving

Ingredients

- 1 tsp each cumin seeds & coriander/cilantro seeds
- 1 tbsp vegetable oil
- 2 garlic cloves, crushed
- ½ tsp chilli powder
- 600g/1lb 5oz raw king prawns, shelled
- 120ml/½ cup low fat crème fraiche
- 4 tbsp tomato puree/paste
- ½ tsp salt
- 2 tbsp freshly chopped coriander/cilantro

Method

1 Quickly cook the cumin & coriander seeds in a dry pan on a medium heat for about 60 seconds. When you begin to smell the aroma remove from the pan and smash with a pestle and mortar.

2 Meanwhile heat the oil in a large non-stick frying pan or wok and sauté the garlic for a minute or two.

3 Add the smashed seeds along with the chilli powder and prawns to the pan. Combine well and cook for 2-3 minutes. Stir through the crème fraiche, tomato puree & salt and gently simmer for 3-5 minutes or until the prawns are pink and cooked though.

4 Sprinkle with chopped coriander and serve.

CHEFS NOTE

Serve with plain boiled rice or stuffed into pitta breads.

BENGALI GRILLED FISH

SERVES 4

230 calories per serving

Ingredients

- 4 large boneless white fish fillets (each weighing 150g/5oz)
- 8 garlic cloves
- 2 large bunches fresh coriander/cilantro
- 2 tbsp mustard oil
- 2 tbsp lemon juice
- 2 tbsp water
- 1 tsp chilli powder
- ½ tsp salt
- 200g/7oz rocket leaves

Method

1 Preheat the grill to a medium high heat.

2 Place the garlic, fresh coriander, oil, lemon juice, water, chilli powder & salt in a food processor and pulse until finely chopped into a paste (add a little more water if you need to loosen it up).

3 Cover the fish fillets with the paste and grill for 8-12 minutes or until cooked through.

4 Season and serve with the rocket leaves on the side.

CHEFS NOTE

This is a super easy light lunch, bulk it up with a veggie side dish or rice for dinner.

SERVES 4

TAMARIND PRAWNS

275
calories per serving

Ingredients

- 1 tsp each cumin seeds & coriander/ cilantro seeds
- ½ tsp chilli powder
- 2 garlic cloves, crushed
- 4 tbsp water
- 2 red peppers, deseeded & sliced
- 2 tsp vegetable oil
- 1 onion, peeled & sliced
- 600g/1lb 5oz raw king prawns. Shelled
- 1 tbsp tamarind paste
- 1 tbsp brown sugar
- ½ tsp salt
- 2 tbsp freshly chopped coriander/ cilantro

Method

1 Use a pestle and mortar to grind down the cumin & coriander seeds. Add the chilli powder, crushed garlic & water to make a paste.

2 Meanwhile heat the oil in a large non-stick frying pan or wok and sauté the onions & peppers for a few minutes until they begin to soften.

3 Add the spice paste, stir well and cook for 5 minutes. Add the prawns, tamarind paste, sugar & salt and cook for 6-10 minutes or until the prawns are pink and cooked through.

4 Sprinkle with chopped coriander and serve.

CHEFS NOTE

Serve with lemon wedges and flat bread/ rice or salad.

GREAT FOOD EXPRESS QUICK & EASY

Skinny CURRY

VEGETABLE DISHES

SERVES 4

SQUASH & SPINACH ROGAN

190 calories per serving

Ingredients

- 1 tsp cumin seeds
- 4 tbsp fat free Greek yogurt
- 2 tbsp tomato puree/paste
- ½ tsp each ground ginger, chilli powder & turmeric
- 1 tbsp vegetable oil
- 800g/1¾lbs butternut squash peeled & cubed
- 250ml/1 cup vegetable stock or water
- 150g/5oz spinach

Method

1 Quickly cook the cumin seeds in a dry non-stick frying pan or wok on a medium heat for about 60 seconds. When you begin to smell the aroma remove from the pan and smash with a pestle and mortar.

2 Mix these crushed seeds with the Greek yoghurt, tomato puree, ginger, chilli powder & turmeric.

3 Meanwhile heat the oil in the non-stick frying pan before adding the cubed squash and stir-frying for 5 minutes. Stir through the spiced yogurt and combine for a minute.

4 Add the stock, cover and increase the heat. Cook for about 5-10 minutes, or until the stock has evaporated and the squash is tender.

5 Stir through the spinach and serve.

CHEFS NOTE

Cook for a couple of minutes longer if you want the spinach to be wilted.

SERVES 4

PANEER & PEPPER KEBABS

350 calories per serving

Ingredients

- 2 red peppers
- 1 red onion
- 1 tsp salt
- 2 tsp vegetable oil
- 4 garlic cloves, crushed
- 2 tsp freshly grated ginger
- 1 tsp each chilli powder, coriander/ cilantro & cumin
- 2 tbsp fat free Greek yogurt
- 300g/11oz paneer
- 4 metal skewers
- Lime wedges

Method

1 Preheat the grill to a medium high heat.

2 Deseed the peppers and cut into bite-size chunks. Peel the red onion and do the same with this. Add both these to a bowl and mix with the salt and vegetable oil.

3 Meanwhile mix the garlic, ginger, chilli powder, coriander, cumin & yogurt together.

4 Cut the paneer into bite-size chunks and smother with the yoghurt mixture (if you have the time you could prepare this dish and leave to marinade overnight before cooking).

5 Thread the cubed paneer, peppers & onion pieces in turn onto the skewers. Place the skewers under the grill and cook for 4-5 minutes each side or until everything is cooked through.

6 Season and serve with lime wedges.

CHEFS NOTE

If you find it difficult to source Indian paneer try substituting with tofu.

SERVES 4

VEGETABLE KARALA AVIAL

310 calories per serving

Ingredients

- 1 tsp turmeric
- 250g/9oz cauliflower florets
- 250g/9oz carrots, peeled & cut into batons
- 300g/11oz sweet potatoes, peeled & diced
- 200g/7oz peas
- 200g/7oz green beans
- 1 tbsp vegetable oil
- 2 onions, peeled & sliced
- 3 garlic cloves, crushed
- 1 tsp freshly grated ginger
- 4 curry leaves
- 1 red chilli, deseeded & finely sliced
- 250ml/1 cup low fat coconut milk
- 2 tbsp fat free Greek yogurt
- 3 tbsp freshly chopped coriander/cilantro

Method

1 Bring a pan of salted water to the boil, add the turmeric and cook the vegetables for 5 minutes (not the onions). Drain and put to one side.

2 Meanwhile heat the oil in a large non-stick frying pan or wok and sauté the onions, garlic, ginger, curry leaves and sliced chilli for a few minutes until the onions begin to soften.

3 Add the coconut milk & yoghurt and combine well for a minute or two. Add the cooked vegetables and cook for 4-6 minutes or until the vegetables are tender and to your liking.

CHEFS NOTE

Use whichever mix of vegetables you prefer for this simple veggie dish.

SERVES 4

YOGURT SPICED POTATOES

170 calories per serving

Ingredients

- 800g/1¾lbs potatoes, peeled & cubed
- 1 tsp each cumin seeds & coriander/cilantro seeds
- 4 tbsp fat free Greek yoghurt
- ½ tsp each turmeric, chilli powder, salt, ground ginger & paprika
- 2 tbsp freshly chopped coriander/cilantro

Method

1 Bring a pan of salted water to the boil and cook the potatoes for about 5-6 minutes, or until just tender enough to eat. Drain and put to one side.

2 Meanwhile quickly cook the cumin & coriander seeds in a dry non-stick frying pan or wok on a medium heat for about 60 seconds. When you begin to smell the aroma remove from the pan and smash with a pestle and mortar.

3 Mix these crushed seeds with the Greek yoghurt, turmeric, chilli powder, salt & ginger. Gently heat this mix in the non-stick frying pan before adding the cooked potatoes. Combine well and warm through.

4 Serve with the paprika sprinkled over the top along with the fresh coriander.

CHEFS NOTE

Room temperature yogurt is best for this recipe to prevent the sauce from splitting.

SERVES 4

ALOO PALAK

220 calories per serving

Ingredients

- 800g/1¾lbs potatoes, peeled & cubed
- 1 tsp mustard seeds
- 1 tbsp vegetable oil
- 2 garlic cloves, crushed
- 1 green chilli, deseeded & finely chopped
- ½ tsp each cumin & ground ginger
- 200g/7oz fresh tomatoes, roughly chopped
- 150g/5oz spinach leaves

Method

1 Bring a pan of salted water to the boil and cook the potatoes for about 5-6 minutes, or until just tender enough to eat. Drain and put to one side.

2 Meanwhile heat the oil in a dry non-stick frying pan or wok and heat the mustard seeds for a minute until they begin to pop. Add the garlic & chilli and sauté for a couple of minutes. Add the ground spices & potatoes and stir-fry for 2-3 minutes.

3 Tip in the tomatoes & spinach and stir-fry on a high heat for 2-3 minutes or until everything is piping hot and cooked through (add a splash of water to the pan if you need to loosen it up).

CHEFS NOTE

Serve with plain boiled rice and chutney.

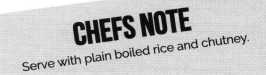

PULAO

SERVES 4

265 calories per serving

Ingredients

- 1 tsp vegetable oil
- 1 onion, peeled & sliced
- 2 garlic cloves, crushed
- 1 tsp freshly grated ginger
- ½ tsp each salt, cumin & chilli powder
- 1 tsp ground coriander/cilantro
- 400g/14oz potatoes, quartered
- 200g/7oz cauliflower florets
- 200g/7oz peas
- 125g/4oz basmati rice
- 500ml/2 cups vegetable stock or water

Method

1 Heat the oil in a large non-stick frying pan or wok and sauté the onions, garlic & ginger for a few minutes until the onions begin to soften (add a splash of water to the pan if needed).

2 Add the salt, cumin, chilli powder & ground coriander and cook for a minute or two.

3 Add the rest of the ingredients to the pan and simmer for 20 minutes or until the rice is tender (add more stock to the rice if needed).

4 Season with a little more salt and serve in shallow bowls.

CHEFS NOTE

This is good served with a garnish of diced cucumber and fresh tomatoes piled on top.

SERVES 4

STREET FOOD VEGGIE CURRY

215 calories per serving

Ingredients

- 1 tbsp vegetable oil
- 2 onions, peeled & sliced
- 2 garlic cloves, crushed
- ½ tsp freshly grated ginger
- ½ tsp each salt, turmeric & chilli powder
- 1 tsp each mango powder, cumin seeds & ground coriander/cilantro
- 250g/9oz cherry tomatoes, quartered
- 250g/9oz carrots, peeled & diced
- 300g/11oz potatoes, peeled & diced
- 200g/7oz peas
- 200g/7oz green beans
- 500ml/2 cups vegetable stock or water
- 3 tbsp freshly chopped coriander/ cilantro

Method

1 Heat the oil in a large non-stick frying pan or wok and sauté the onions, garlic & ginger for a few minutes until the onions begin to soften.

2 Add the salt, turmeric, chilli powder, mango powder, cumin seeds, ground coriander & tomatoes. Stir well before adding the vegetables and stock.

3 Cover the pan, whack up the heat and cook for 8-10 minutes to bind the curry together.

4 Season with a little more salt if needed and serve sprinkled with chopped coriander.

CHEFS NOTE

Popular nationwide as street food, this simple curry is often served loaded into Indian bread rolls

SERVES 4

CHICKPEA CHAAT

300 calories per serving

Ingredients

- 1 tbsp vegetable oil
- 1 onion, peeled & sliced
- 2 garlic cloves, crushed
- 2 green chillies, deseeded & finely chopped
- 1 tsp each salt, cumin seeds & ground coriander/cilantro
- 2 tsp tamarind paste
- 800g/1¾lbs tinned chickpeas, rinsed
- 4 tbsp fat free Greek yoghurt
- 2 tbsp freshly chopped flat leaf parsley

Method

1 Heat the oil in a large non-stick frying pan or wok and add the onion, garlic, green chillies, salt, cumin seeds & ground coriander

2 Stir through the tamarind paste & chickpeas and cook for 5-7 minutes or until the chickpeas are piping hot (add a little water to the pan if you need to keep it loose).

3 Stir through the yoghurt, sprinkle with flat leaf parsley and serve.

CHEFS NOTE

This is good served with lemon wedges on the side

SERVES 4

SIMPLE WARM INDIAN POTATO 'SALAD'

250 calories per serving

Ingredients

- 1 tbsp vegetable oil
- 2 white onions, peeled & sliced
- 800g/1¾lbs potatoes, peeled & cubed
- 1 tsp each mustard seeds, salt & cumin seeds
- 2 red chillies, deseeded & finely chopped
- ½ red onion, peeled & finely sliced

Method

1 Heat the oil in a large non-stick frying pan or wok and add the white onion, potatoes, mustard seeds, salt, cumin seeds & chillies, salt.

2 Sauté for 10-15 minutes or until the potatoes are tender (add a splash of water to the pan every now and again if needed).

3 Serve with red onion sprinkled over the top.

CHEFS NOTE

Cube the potatoes to about 2cm in size so that they cook quickly and evenly.

SERVES 4

CRUSHED PANEER STIR-FRY

260 calories per serving

Ingredients

- 1 tbsp vegetable oil
- 2 onions, peeled & sliced
- 1 green chilli, deseeded & finely chopped
- ½ tsp each salt & brown sugar
- 1 tsp each cumin seeds & turmeric
- 300g/11oz cherry tomatoes, halved
- 200g/7oz paneer, cubed
- 2 tbsp freshly chopped coriander/ cilantro

Method

1 Heat the oil in a large non-stick frying pan or wok and add the onions, chillies, salt, sugar, cumin seeds & turmeric.

2 Sauté for 5 minutes and add the tomatoes. Stir-fry for a further 5 minutes and throw in the cubed paneer. As the cheese cooks smash it up a little with a wooden spoon and when everything is piping hot stir through the fresh coriander.

3 Check the seasoning and serve.

CHEFS NOTE

Quick and easy this makes a tasty lunch or supper.

SERVES 4

SPICY DRESSED BEANS

200 calories per serving

Ingredients

- 1 tsp each ground cumin & fresh oregano
- ½ tsp salt
- 1 red chilli, deseeded & finely chopped
- 2 tbsp lemon juice
- 1 red onion, peeled & finely chopped
- 1 cucumber, finely diced
- 600g/1lb 5oz tinned mixed beans, rinsed
- 200g/7oz cherry tomatoes, halved
- 2 tbsp freshly chopped flat leaf parsley

Method

1 Quickly cook the cumin seeds in a dry non-stick pan on a medium heat for about 60 seconds. When you begin to smell the aroma remove from the pan and smash with a pestle and mortar.

2 Combine all the ingredients together in a large bowl tossing everything well to ensure good overage.

3 Check the balance of salt & lemon juice, adjusting according to your own taste.

4 Pile into bowls and serve as a super fast salad lunch.

CHEFS NOTE

Served with green leaves or fresh baby spinach leaves this makes a refreshing, light meal.

SERVES 4

CUCUMBER & MUSTARD SEED DHAL

180 calories per serving

Ingredients

- 150g/5oz split yellow lentils, rinsed
- 370ml/1½ cups vegetable stock or water
- ½ tsp turmeric
- 1 cucumber, cut into batons
- 1 tsp vegetable oil
- 2 garlic cloves, crushed
- 1 tsp mustard seeds
- 1 red chilli, deseeded & finely chopped
- ½ tsp salt

Method

1 Add the lentils, stock & turmeric to a saucepan and bring to the boil. Reduce the heat to a simmer and cook for 20-25 minutes or until the lentils are tender and turn into a thick paste (add more stock if needed throughout this process and remove any scum which floats to the top of the pan).

2 When the lentils are just ready add the cucumber pieces and stir through.

3 Meanwhile heat the oil in a non-stick frying pan and quickly add the garlic, mustard seeds, sliced chilli and salt (add a splash of water to the pan if needed). Cook for 60 seconds on a high heat add to the lentil pan and stir through.

4 Divide into bowls and serve.

CHEFS NOTE

Perfect for summer, the cucumber in this dhal adds a refreshing crisp crunch.

SERVES 4

AROMATIC KIDNEY BEAN CURRY

320 calories per serving

Ingredients

- 1 tbsp vegetable oil
- 4 green cardamoms
- 2 cloves
- 1 tsp cumin seeds
- 1 onion, peeled & sliced
- 1 garlic clove, crushed
- 1 tsp each freshly grated ginger & ground coriander
- 800g/1¾lbs tinned chopped tomatoes
- 800g/1¾lbs tinned kidney beans, rinsed
- ½ tsp each salt, chilli powder & ground cinnamon

Method

1 Heat the oil in a large non-stick frying pan or wok and add the cardamoms, cloves & cumin seeds. Cook for a minute before adding the cumin seeds, onion, garlic, ginger & ground coriander.

2 Simmer on a medium heat for 2-3 minutes and add the chopped tomatoes, kidney beans, salt, chilli powder and ground cinnamon.

3 Carry on cooking for 10 minutes or until the beans are cooked through. Check the seasoning and serve.

CHEFS NOTE

Mash a handful of the cooked kidney beans with the back of a fork to bind the curry together.

SERVES 4

SPICED CHICKPEAS

285 calories per serving

Ingredients

- 1 tbsp vegetable oil
- 1 onion, peeled & sliced
- 2 garlic cloves, crushed
- 1 tsp each freshly grated ginger, ground coriander/cilantro, cumin & chilli powder
- 400g/14oz fresh vine-ripened tomatoes, roughly chopped
- 1 tbsp tomato puree/paste
- 150g/5oz spinach
- 800g/1¾lbs tinned chickpeas beans, rinsed
- 2 tbsp freshly chopped coriander/ cilantro

Method

1 Heat the oil in a large non-stick frying pan or wok and add the onion, garlic, ginger, ground coriander, cumin & chilli powder.

2 Simmer on a medium heat for 2-3 minutes then add the fresh chopped tomatoes and puree. Cook for 5 minutes before adding the spinach and chickpeas.

3 Carry on cooking for 10 minutes or until the beans are cooked through (add a splash of water to the pan occasionally if you need to). Check the seasoning and serve with the fresh coriander sprinkled over the top.

CHEFS NOTE

You could use freshly chopped flat leaf parsley in place of fresh coriander if you wish.

SERVES 4

RED ONION DHAL

180 calories per serving

Ingredients

- 150g/5oz split yellow lentils, rinsed
- 370ml/1½ cups vegetable stock or water
- ½ tsp turmeric
- 1 tsp vegetable oil
- 1 red onion, peeled & sliced
- 4 garlic cloves, crushed
- 1 tsp cumin seeds
- 1 green chilli, deseeded & finely chopped
- 125g/4oz spinach leaves
- 1 tbsp lemon juice

Method

1 Add the lentils, stock & turmeric to a saucepan and bring to the boil. Reduce the heat to a simmer and cook for 20-25 minutes or until the lentils are tender and turn into a thick paste (add more stock if needed throughout this process and remove any scum which floats to the top of the pan).

2 When the lentils are ready heat the oil in a non-stick frying pan and quickly add the onion, garlic, cumin seeds, chopped chilli & spinach leaves (add a splash of water to the pan if needed). Cook for two minutes, add to the lentil pan and stir through along with the lemon juice.

3 Check the seasoning, divide into bowls and serve.

CHEFS NOTE

You could also add some thinly sliced raw red onion to this dhal as a garnish.

SERVES 4

PUNJABI MATAR PANEER

340 calories per serving

Ingredients

- 1 tsp vegetable oil
- 250g/9oz paneer cheese, cubed
- 2 onions, peeled & sliced
- 3 garlic cloves, crushed
- 2 tsp freshly grated ginger
- 250g/9oz vine-ripened tomatoes, roughly chopped
- ½ tsp each ground black pepper, salt, turmeric & chilli powder
- 1 tsp each ground coriander/cilantro, cumin
- 200g/7oz frozen peas
- 150g/5oz spinach leaves
- 1 red chilli, deseeded & finely chopped
- 4 tbsp fat free Greek yogurt
- 2 tbsp freshly chopped coriander/cilantro

Method

1 Heat the oil in a large non-stick frying pan or wok and quickly fry the paneer cubes for a minute each side until golden brown. Remove these to a plate and add the onions, garlic & ginger to the pan. Sauté on a medium heat for a few minutes until the onions begin to soften.

2 Add the chopped tomatoes, pepper, salt, turmeric, chilli powder, ground coriander, cumin & peas and move around the pan for 10 minutes or until the tomatoes begin to disintegrate (add a splash of water to the pan if you find the spices are sticking to the pan).

3 Add the spinach, chopped chilli & yoghurt and cook for a further 5 minutes. Add the browned paneer cubes and cook for 4-6minutes or until everything is piping hot and cooked through.

CHEFS NOTE

Paneer cheese is now widely available, cut into bite sized cubes for this recipe. You could try substituting with tofu fi you find paneer difficult to source.

SERVES 4

CUMIN & GARLIC DHAL

165 calories per serving

Ingredients

- 150g/5oz split yellow lentils, rinsed
- 370ml/1½ cups vegetable stock or water
- ½ tsp turmeric
- 1 tsp vegetable oil
- 4 garlic cloves, crushed
- 1 tsp cumin seeds
- ½ tsp chilli powder
- 1 red chilli, deseeded & finely chopped
- 1 tsp salt

Method

1 Add the lentils, stock & turmeric to a saucepan and bring to the boil. Reduce the heat to a simmer and cook for 20-25 minutes or until the lentils are tender and turn into a thick paste (add more stock if needed throughout this process and remove any scum which floats to the top of the pan).

2 When the lentils are ready heat the oil in a non-stick frying pan and quickly add the garlic, cumin seeds, chilli powder, sliced chilli and salt (add a splash of water to the pan if needed). Cook for two minutes, add to the lentil pan and stir through.

3 Divide into bowls and serve.

CHEFS NOTE

This is a simple dhal, which can be served with roti as a main course.

SERVES 4

RED LENTIL DHAL

300 calories per serving

Ingredients

- 200g/7oz split yellow lentils, rinsed
- 500ml/2 cups vegetable stock or water
- ½ tsp turmeric
- 200g/7oz carrots, finely diced
- 200g/7oz frozen peas
- 1 tbsp vegetable oil
- 4 garlic cloves, crushed
- 1 tsp cumin seeds
- 2 green chillies, deseeded & finely chopped
- 1 tsp salt

Method

1 Add the lentils, stock & turmeric to a saucepan and bring to the boil. Reduce the heat to a simmer and cook for 20 minutes or until the lentils are tender and turn into a thick paste (add more stock if needed throughout this process and remove any scum which floats to the top of the pan).

2 Add the carrots & peas to the pan and continue to cook. Meanwhile heat the oil in a non-stick frying pan and quickly add the garlic, cumin seeds, sliced chillies and salt (add a splash of water to the pan if needed). Cook for 2-3 minutes, add to the lentil pan and stir through.

3 Divide into bowls and serve.

CHEFS NOTE

Serve on a bed of rice or green salad leaves for a comforting and quick veggie meal.

GREAT FOOD EXPRESS QUICK & EASY

Skinny

CURRY

VEGETABLE SIDES

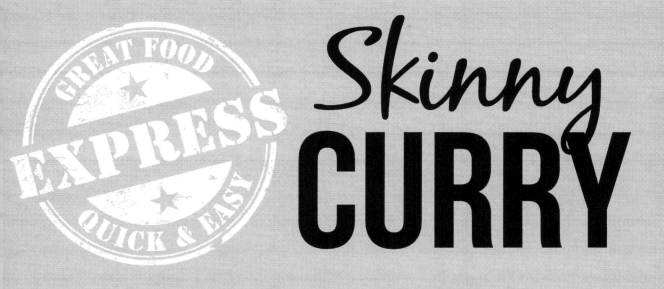

ALOO GOBI

SERVES 4

150 calories per serving

Ingredients

- 1 tbsp vegetable oil
- 1 onion, peeled & sliced
- 2 garlic cloves, crushed
- ½ tsp freshly grated ginger
- 400g/14oz potatoes, quartered
- ½ tsp each salt, turmeric & chilli powder
- 1 tsp each ground coriander/cilantro & cumin
- 400g/14oz cauliflower florets (bite sized)
- 1 tsp garam masala
- 3 tbsp freshly chopped coriander/ cilantro

Method

1 Heat the oil in a large non-stick frying pan or wok and sauté the onions, garlic & ginger for a few minutes until the onions begin to soften.

2 Add the potatoes, salt, turmeric, chilli powder, ground coriander & cumin along with a splash of water. Cover and cook for 5-7 minutes or until the potatoes are on their way to being tender.

3 Add the bite sized cauliflower florets, stir well and cook for a further 5 minutes or until the potatoes and cauliflower are tender (but not soft).

4 Sprinkle with garam masala, season with a little more salt if needed and serve sprinkled with chopped coriander.

CHEFS NOTE

Simple and delicious this dish is good with a salad or served with Indian bread.

SPINACH PANEER

SERVES 4

200 calories per serving

Ingredients

- 1 tsp vegetable oil
- 250g/9oz paneer cheese, cubed
- 1 green chilli, deseeded & sliced
- 2 onions, peeled & sliced
- 2 garlic cloves, crushed
- 2 tsp freshly grated ginger
- 1 tsp each salt & cumin
- 600g/1lb 5oz spinach leaves
- 120ml/½ cup hot water

Method

1 Heat the oil in a large non-stick frying pan or wok and quickly fry the paneer cubes for a minute each side until golden brown. Remove these to a plate and add the chopped chillies, onions, garlic & ginger to the pan. Sauté on a medium heat for a few minutes until the onions begin to soften.

2 Add the salt, cumin, spinach leaves & hot water and cook for 5 minutes or until the spinach has wilted. Tip the contents of the frying pan into a blender and blend until smooth. Add a little more hot water to the blender if needed to make a thick soup-like paste.

3 Tip the spinach puree back into the frying pan, add the browned paneer cubes and cook for 10 minutes or until everything is piping hot and cooked through.

CHEFS NOTE

Serve as a veggie side or with warm naan as a tasty main course.

COCONUT CORN

SERVES 4

110 calories per serving

Ingredients

- 1 tbsp vegetable oil
- 1 tsp each cumin seeds & mustard seeds
- 1 red chilli, deseeded & finely chopped
- ½ tsp each chilli powder, mango powder, turmeric & coriander/cilantro
- 400g/14oz frozen sweetcorn
- 250ml/1 cup low fat coconut milk

Method

1. Heat the oil in the non-stick frying pan and add the cumin seeds & mustard seeds. After a minute or two the mustard seeds will begin to pop.
2. Add the sliced chilli and dried spices to the pan and cook for 2 minutes (add a splash of water if you need to loosen it up).
3. Add the sweetcorn and stir-fry for 5 minutes. Pour in the coconut milk and gently simmer for 2-3 minutes or until the corn is tender and the coconut milk is piping hot.

CHEFS NOTE

Double the quantities and add a handful of asparagus or green beans to turn this into a veggie main course.

SERVES 4

MUSTARD SEED ASPARAGUS

160 calories per serving

Ingredients

- 1 tsp mustard seeds
- ½ tsp cumin seeds
- 1 tbsp vegetable oil
- 400g/14oz asparagus tips
- ½ tsp each chilli powder, ground ginger & salt

Method

1 Heat the oil in a dry non-stick frying pan or wok and add the mustard seeds & cumin seeds. After a minute or two the mustard seeds will begin to pop.

2 Add the asparagus tips, chilli powder, ginger & salt and stir-fry on a high heat for 3-4 minutes or until the asparagus is cooked to your liking (add a splash of water to the pan if you need to loosen it up).

CHEFS NOTE

This is a simple dry side dish, which can be served in place of rice or bread.

SERVES 4

SPICED BAKED AUBERGINE & TOMATOES

220 calories per serving

Ingredients

- 2 large aubergines/egg plant, cubed
- 1 tsp each turmeric & chilli powder
- ½ tsp salt
- 1 tbsp vegetable oil
- 2 tsp fennel seeds
- 1 tsp cumin seeds
- 2 tsp dried oregano or thyme
- 400g/14oz tinned chopped tomatoes

Method

1 Preheat the oven to 220C/425F/Gas 7.

2 Mix together the cubed aubergine with the turmeric, chilli powder & salt.

3 Meanwhile combine the oil in a shallow ovenproof dish along with the fennel seeds, cumin seeds & dried oregano (or thyme). Pop this in the oven and leave to warm for a couple of minutes.

4 After this time stir the cubed aubergine into the warmed oil and add the chopped tomatoes.

5 Return to the oven and cook for 30 minutes or until everything is piping hot and cooked though.

6 Divide into bowls and serve with lots of green vegetables or Indian bread.

CHEFS NOTE

This takes a little longer to cook than some of the other express recipes but it is super simple to make.

SERVES 4

STIR-FRIED MUSHROOMS & FRESH CORIANDER

120 calories per serving

Ingredients

- 1 tsp each cumin seeds & coriander/ cilantro seeds
- 1 tsp vegetable oil
- 2 garlic cloves, crushed
- 1 tsp freshly grated ginger
- 1 onion, sliced
- 2 green chillies, deseeded & very finely sliced
- 500g/1lb 2oz mushrooms, halved
- 300g/11oz tomatoes, roughly chopped
- ½ tsp salt
- 2 tbsp freshly chopped coriander/ cilantro

Method

1 Quickly cook the cumin & coriander seeds in a dry non-stick frying pan or wok on a medium heat for about 60 seconds. When you begin to smell the aroma remove from the pan and smash with a pestle and mortar.

2 Heat the oil in the same pan and gently sauté the garlic, ginger, onions & chillies for a few minutes until the onions soften.

3 Put the smashed seeds back into the pan, add the mushrooms, tomatoes & salt and stir-fry on a medium heat for 5 minutes.

4 Increase the heat to boil off any excess liquid and serve with more salt if needed and coriander sprinkled over the top.

CHEFS NOTE

Use any type of closed cup mushroom you prefer.

GREAT FOOD EXPRESS QUICK & EASY

Skinny CURRY

RICE & BREAD

SERVES 4

PERFECT PLAIN BASMATI RICE

265 calories per serving

Ingredients

- 300g/11oz rice
- 500ml/2 cups water
- ½ tsp lemon juice

PLAIN & SIMPLE

Method

1 Put the rice in a sieve and rinse with running water, then leave it to soak in a bowl of cold water for 20 minutes.

2 Drain and place in a pan with 500ml fresh, cold water. Bring to the boil, add the lemon juice and quickly combine.

3 Cover and leave to simmer for 8-10 minutes or until the rice is tender and the water has been absorbed (keep an eye on it and add a little more water if needed),

4 Remove from the heat. Uncover and leave to stand for a minute or two.

5 Fluff with a fork and serve.

CHEFS NOTE

If you don't have time to soak the rice just rinse it and add straight to the pan.

SERVES 4

SWEET SULTANA RICE

310 calories per serving

Ingredients

- 620ml/2½ cups warm water
- 1 tbsp brown sugar
- 300g/11oz rice
- 2 tbsp sultanas, chopped
- ½ tsp ground cinnamon

Method

1 On a gentle heat combine the sugar and water together in a pan. Add the rice and bring to the boil.

2 Cover and leave to simmer for 8-10 minutes.

3 Add the sultanas & cinnamon, stir once and cook for a further 5 minutes or until the rice is tender and the water has been absorbed (keep an eye on it and add a little more water if needed),

4 Remove from the heat. Uncover and leave to stand for a minute or two.

5 Fluff with a fork and serve.

CHEFS NOTE

You could try adding saffron threads to the pan and garnish this simple sweet rice with chopped nuts.

SERVES 4

AROMATIC PILAU RICE

275 calories per serving

Ingredients

- 300g/11oz rice
- 1 tsp vegetable oil
- 1 onion, sliced
- 4 cardamom pods
- ¼ tsp ground cloves
- 1 cinnamon stick
- 2 bay leaves
- 500ml/2 cups vegetable stock

Method

1 Put the rice in a sieve and rinse with running water, then leave it to soak in a bowl of cold water for 20 minutes.

2 Meanwhile heat the oil in a non-stick lidded frying pan and sauté the onion for a few minutes until softened. Add the cardamom pods, ground cloves, cinnamon stick & bay leaves and combine well.

3 Drain the rice and add this, along with the stock, to the pan. Bring to the boil, cover and leave to simmer for 8-10 minutes or until the rice is tender and the stock has been absorbed (keep an eye on it and add a little more stock if needed).

4 Remove from the heat, uncover and leave to stand for a minute or two.

5 Fluff with a fork and serve.

CHEFS NOTE

Fish out the cinnamon stick & bay leaves before serving.

SERVES 4

MUSHROOM PILAFF

295 calories per serving

Ingredients

- 300g/11oz rice
- 1 tsp vegetable oil
- 1 tsp cumin seeds
- 1 onion, sliced
- 200g/7oz mushrooms, finely chopped
- 2 garlic cloves, crushed
- ½ tsp salt
- 500ml/2 cups vegetable stock

Method

1 Put the rice in a sieve and rinse with running water, then leave it to soak in a bowl of cold water for 20 minutes.

2 Meanwhile heat the oil in a non-stick lidded frying pan and sauté the cumin seeds, onion, mushrooms, garlic & salt for 5 minutes until softened.

3 Drain the rice and add this, along with the stock, to the pan. Bring to the boil, cover and leave to simmer for 8-10 minutes or until the rice is tender and the stock has been absorbed (keep an eye on it and add a little more stock if needed).

4 Remove from the heat, uncover and leave to stand for a minute or two.

5 Fluff with a fork and serve.

CHEFS NOTE

Try serving with some chopped cashew nuts and fresh coriander.

MAKES 10

CHAPATTI BREAD

90
calories per serving

Ingredients

- 250g/9oz flour
- 1 tsp salt
- 2 tbsp vegetable oil
- 120ml/ ½ cup warm water (use more if needed)
- Low cal cooking oil spray

USE WHOLEMEAL FLOUR

Method

1 Combine together the flour, salt, oil and water to make a soft, but not sticky, dough.

2 Knead the dough for a few minutes on a floured surface and divide into 10 balls.

3 Lightly cover and leave for 20 minutes before using a rolling pin to roll each ball out into a flat 'pancake'.

4 Place a non-stick frying pan on a medium heat with a spray of low cal cooking oil. When the pan is nice and hot put the chapatti on it and cook for 30 seconds. Flip and cook for 30 seconds longer

CHEFS NOTE

Super quick and easy to make it makes sense to make a larger batch, which you can store in the freezer.

MAKES 10

SPICED SPINACH CHAPATTI BREAD

100 calories per serving

Ingredients

- 250g/9oz wholemeal flour
- 1 tsp salt
- 1 tsp chilli powder
- 2 tbsp vegetable oil
- 120ml/½ cup warm water (use more if needed)
- 50g/2oz spinach, finely chopped
- Low cal cooking oil spray

Method

1 Combine together the flour, salt, chilli powder, oil and water to make a soft, but not sticky, dough.

2 Add the chopped spinach and knead the dough for a few minutes on a floured surface until the dough is soft and the spinach is well combined into the dough.

3 Divide into 10 balls, gently cover and leave for 20 minutes before using a rolling pin to roll each ball out into a flat 'pancake'.

4 Place a non-stick frying pan on a medium heat with a spray of low cal cooking oil. When the pan is nice and hot put the chapatti on it and cook for 30 seconds. Flip and cook for 30 seconds longer.

CHEFS NOTE

Feel free to experiment with whichever spices you prefer in this simple bread

Skinny CURRY

GREAT FOOD EXPRESS QUICK & EASY

CHUTNEYS & DIPS

SERVES 4

MINTED YOGURT

35 calories per serving

Ingredients

- 1 tbsp freshly chopped mint
- 5 tbsp fat free Greek yogurt
- ½ tsp paprika
- 1 red chilli, deseeded & finely chopped
- ½ tsp salt

COOLING!

Method

Mix all the ingredients together in a small bowl and refrigerate. Or alternatively don't bother chopping the chilli & mint and instead throw everything into a food processor and pulse.

CHEFS NOTE

Super simple, this cooling mint yogurt is great served with really spicy dishes.

SERVES 4

CORIANDER YOGURT CHUTNEY

45 calories per serving

Ingredients

- 1 tsp vegetable oil
- 1 tsp mustard seeds
- Bunch of fresh coriander/cilantro
- 5 tbsp fat free Greek yogurt
- ½ tsp salt

Method

1 Heat the oil in a non-stick frying pan or wok and add the mustard seeds. After a minute or two the mustard seeds will begin to pop.

2 Tip the mustard seeds into a food processor along with all the other ingredients and pulse for a few seconds.

3 Add a little more salt if needed and serve.

CHEFS NOTE

For a more subtle taste, use flat leaf parsley instead of coriander.

SERVES 4

SWEET TOMATO CHUTNEY

45 calories per serving

Ingredients

- 1 tsp vegetable oil
- 1 tsp freshly grated ginger
- 1 red chilli, deseeded & finely chopped
- 1 tbsp raisins
- 300g/11oz fresh tomatoes, chopped
- 1 tbsp brown sugar
- ½ tsp salt

Method

1 Heat the oil in a non-stick frying pan or wok and add the ginger & chopped chillies to sauté for a minute or two.

2 Add the raisins, tomatoes, sugar & salt and cook for 10-15 minutes or until the tomatoes loose their shape. Allow to cool and serve.

CHEFS NOTE

This sweet chutney can be stored in the fridge for up to 3 days.

SERVES 4

COCONUT CHUTNEY

135
calories per serving

Ingredients

- 50g/2oz desiccated coconut
- 200g/7oz fresh tomatoes, chopped
- 1 tsp vegetable oil
- 1 tsp mustard seeds
- 4 curry leaves
- 2 red chillies, deseeded & finely chopped
- ½ tsp salt

Method

1 Rehydrate the coconut in a bowl small of warm water for 10 minutes (use just enough water to cover the coconut).

2 Meanwhile heat the oil in a non-stick frying pan or wok and add the tomatoes, mustard seeds curry leaves, sliced chillies & salt. Sauté for a few minutes, before adding the rehydrated coconut to the pan.

3 Stir well, adjust the seasoning, allow to cool and serve.

CHEFS NOTE

Feel free to put this into a food processor after cooking to get a smoother texture.

SERVES 4

KERALA TOMATO RELISH

45 calories per serving

Ingredients

- 1 red onion
- 250g/5oz fresh ripe tomatoes
- Small bunch of fresh coriander/cilantro
- 1 tbsp lime juice
- ½ tsp each salt & brown sugar

Method

1 Peel and finely dice the onion.

2 Roughly chop the ripe tomatoes and finely chop the fresh coriander.

3 Mix these together along with the lime juice, salt & sugar.

4 Adjust the sugar and salt to suit your taste and serve.

CHEFS NOTE

Relish and chutney is served with almost every Indian meal.

SERVES 4

QUICK HOT CARROT 'PICKLE'

35 calories per serving

Ingredients

- 2 medium carrots
- 2 green chillies
- 1 tsp vegetable oil
- 1 tsp each mustard seeds & cumin seeds
- ½ tsp each turmeric & salt
- 120ml/ ½ cup water

Method

1 Peel the carrots and cut into batons.

2 Deseed the chillies and cut into long, lengthways slices.

3 Meanwhile heat the oil in a non-stick frying pan or wok and add the mustard & cumin seeds. Cook for about 60 seconds before adding the carrots, chillies, turmeric and salt. Stir-fry for 2 minutes and add the water.

4 Simmer for 5-6 minutes or until the water disappears and the carrots are tender. Tip into a bowl and serve straightaway.

CHEFS NOTE

This type of vegetable 'pickle' is a commonplace addition to many Indian meals.

CUCUMBER RAITA

SERVES 4

45 calories per serving

Ingredients

- ½ cucumber
- Small bunch of mint
- 5 tbsp fat free Greek yogurt
- ½ tsp salt

TRY CORIANDER

Method

1 First peel the cucumber and coarsely grate the flesh.

2 Remove any tough mint stalks and finely chop the leaves.

3 Mix all the ingredients together in a small bowl, cover and refrigerate.

CHEFS NOTE

This cooling raita is best served straight away but it can 'keep' in the fridge for up to 2 days. Just give it a good stir through first.

CONVERSION CHART: DRY INGREDIENTS

Metric	Imperial
7g	¼ oz
15g	½ oz
20g	¾ oz
25g	1 oz
40g	1½oz
50g	2oz
60g	2½oz
75g	3oz
100g	3½oz
125g	4oz
140g	4½oz
150g	5oz
165g	5½oz
175g	6oz
200g	7oz
225g	8oz
250g	9oz
275g	10oz
300g	11oz
350g	12oz
375g	13oz
400g	14oz

Metric	Imperial
425g	15oz
450g	1lb
500g	1lb 2oz
550g	1¼lb
600g	1lb 5oz
650g	1lb 7oz
675g	1½lb
700g	1lb 9oz
750g	1lb 11oz
800g	1¾lb
900g	2lb
1kg	2¼lb
1.1kg	2½lb
1.25kg	2¾lb
1.35kg	3lb
1.5kg	3lb 6oz
1.8kg	4lb
2kg	4½lb
2.25kg	5lb
2.5kg	5½lb
2.75kg	6lb

CONVERSION CHART: LIQUID MEASURES

Metric	Imperial	US
25ml	1fl oz	
60ml	2fl oz	¼ cup
75ml	2½ fl oz	
100ml	3½fl oz	
120ml	4fl oz	½ cup
150ml	5fl oz	
175ml	6fl oz	
200ml	7fl oz	
250ml	8½ fl oz	1 cup
300ml	10½ fl oz	
360ml	12½ fl oz	
400ml	14fl oz	
450ml	15½ fl oz	
600ml	1 pint	
750ml	1¼ pint	3 cups
1 litre	1½ pints	4 cups

Other COOKNATION TITLES

If you enjoyed 'The Skinny Express Curry Recipe Book' we'd really appreciate your feedback. Reviews help others decide if this is the right book for them so a moment of your time would be appreciated.

Thank you.

You may also be interested in other '**Skinny**' titles in the CookNation series. You can find all the following great titles by searching under '**CookNation**'.

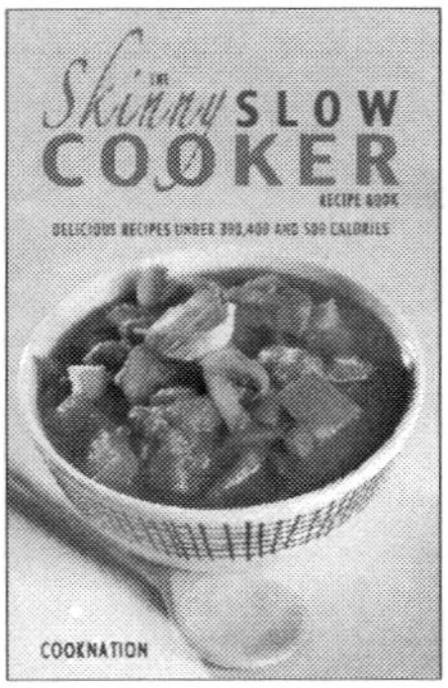

THE SKINNY SLOW COOKER RECIPE BOOK

Delicious Recipes Under 300, 400 And 500 Calories.

Paperback / eBook

THE SKINNY INDIAN TAKEAWAY RECIPE BOOK

Authentic British Indian Restaurant Dishes Under 300, 400 And 500 Calories. The Secret To Low Calorie Indian Takeaway Food At Home.

Paperback / eBook

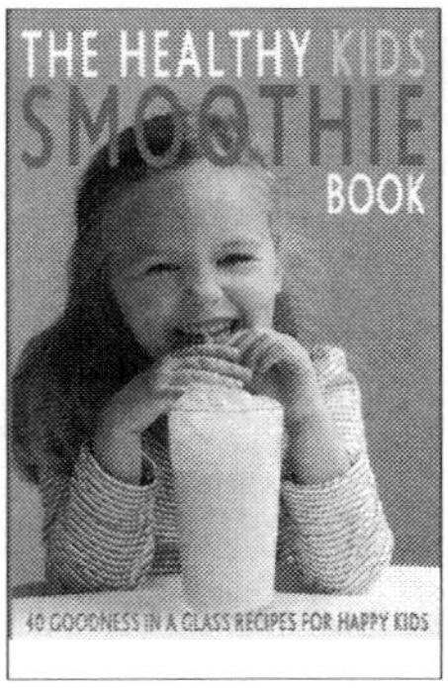

THE HEALTHY KIDS SMOOTHIE BOOK

40 Delicious Goodness In A Glass Recipes for Happy Kids.

eBook

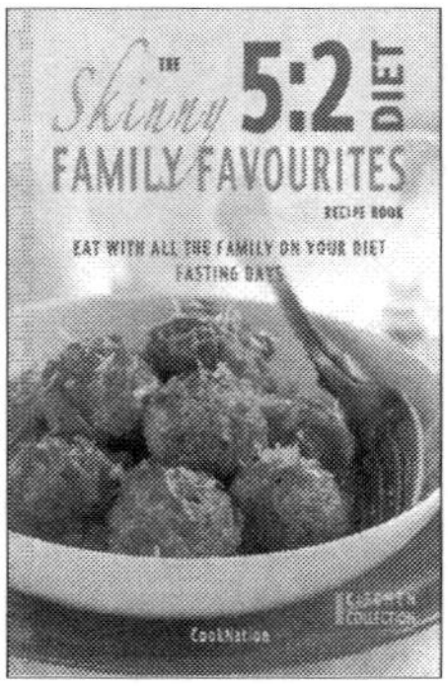

THE SKINNY 5:2 FAST DIET FAMILY FAVOURITES RECIPE BOOK

Eat With All The Family On Your Diet Fasting Days.

Paperback / eBook

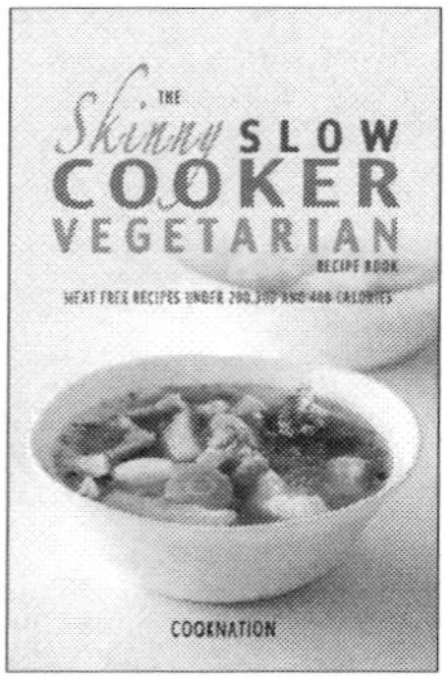

THE SKINNY SLOW COOKER VEGETARIAN RECIPE BOOK

40 Delicious Recipes Under 200, 300 And 400 Calories.

Paperback / eBook

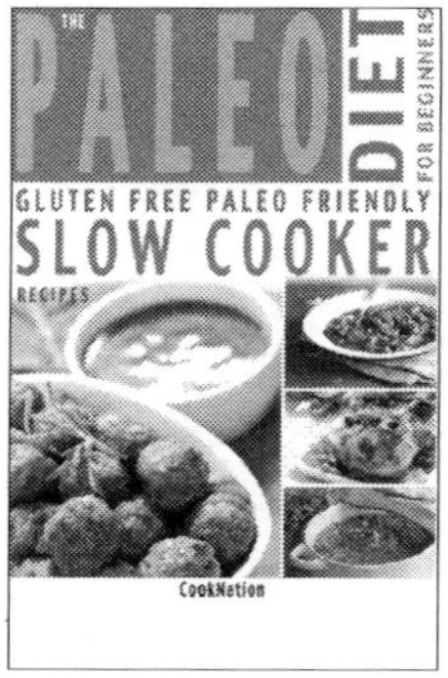

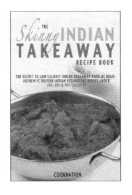

THE PALEO DIET FOR BEGINNERS SLOW COOKER RECIPE BOOK

Gluten Free, Everyday Essential Slow Cooker Paleo Recipes For Beginners.

eBook

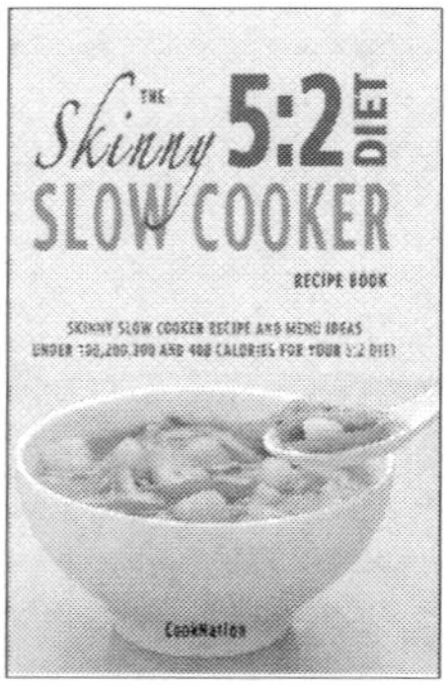

THE SKINNY 5:2 SLOW COOKER RECIPE BOOK

Skinny Slow Cooker Recipe And Menu Ideas Under 100, 200, 300 & 400 Calories For Your 5:2 Diet.

Paperback / eBook

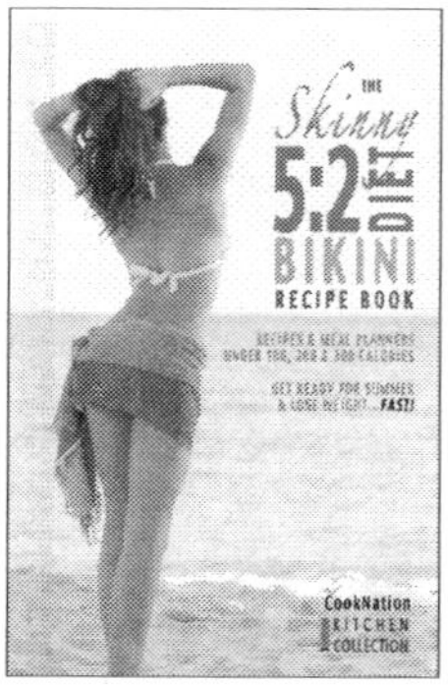

THE SKINNY 5:2 BIKINI DIET RECIPE BOOK

Recipes & Meal Planners Under 100, 200 & 300 Calories. Get Ready For Summer & Lose Weight...FAST!

Paperback / eBook

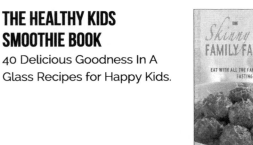

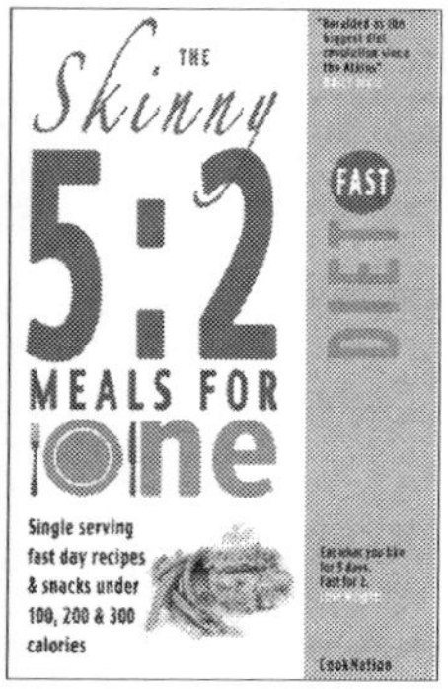

THE SKINNY 5:2 FAST DIET MEALS FOR ONE

Single Serving Fast Day Recipes & Snacks Under 100, 200 & 300 Calories.

Paperback / eBook

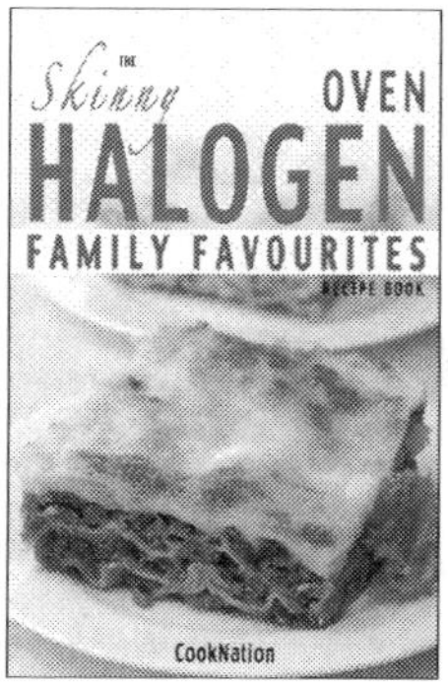

THE SKINNY HALOGEN OVEN FAMILY FAVOURITES RECIPE BOOK

Healthy, Low Calorie Family Meal-Time Halogen Oven Recipes Under 300, 400 and 500 Calories.

Paperback / eBook

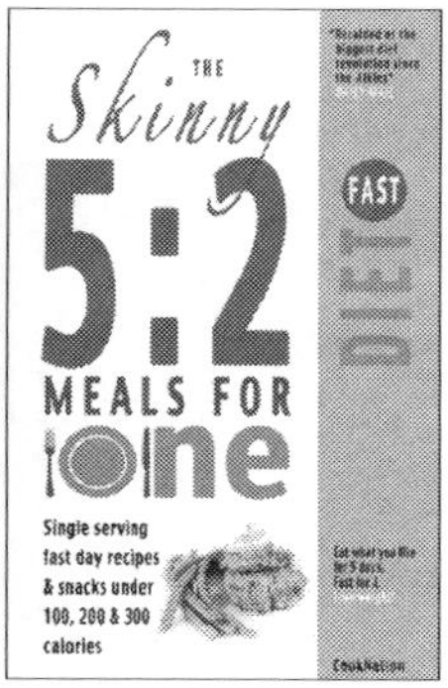

THE SKINNY 5:2 FAST DIET VEGETARIAN MEALS FOR ONE

Single Serving Fast Day Recipes & Snacks Under 100, 200 & 300 Calories.

Paperback / eBook

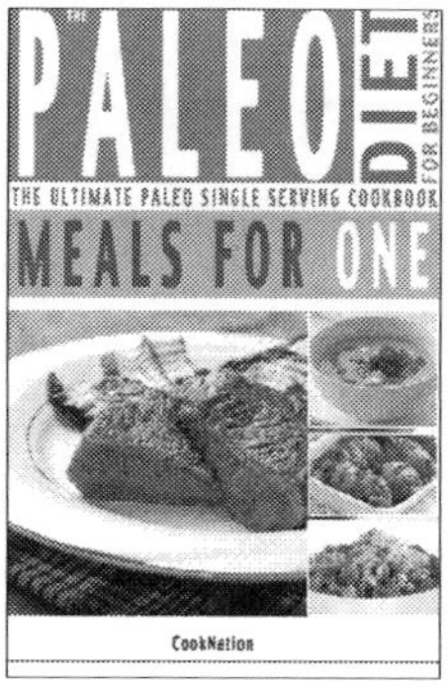

THE PALEO DIET FOR BEGINNERS MEALS FOR ONE

The Ultimate Paleo Single Serving Cookbook.

Paperback / eBook

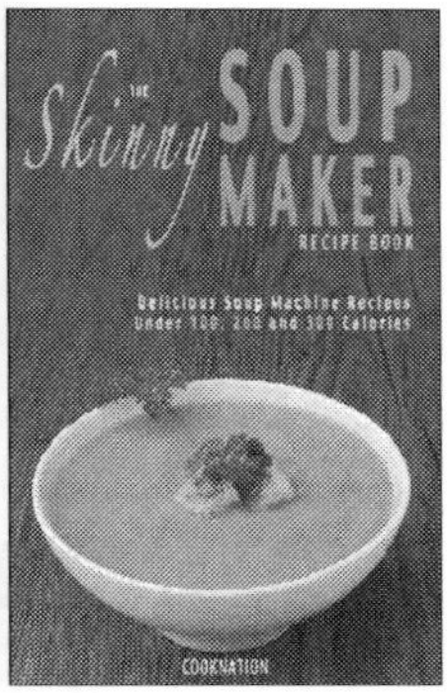

THE SKINNY SOUP MAKER RECIPE BOOK

Delicious Low Calorie, Healthy and Simple Soup Recipes Under 100, 200 and 300 Calories. Perfect For Any Diet and Weight Loss Plan.

Paperback / eBook

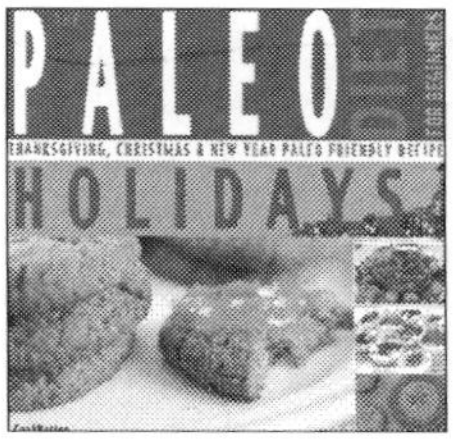

THE PALEO DIET FOR BEGINNERS HOLIDAYS

Thanksgiving, Christmas & New Year Paleo Friendly Recipes.

eBook

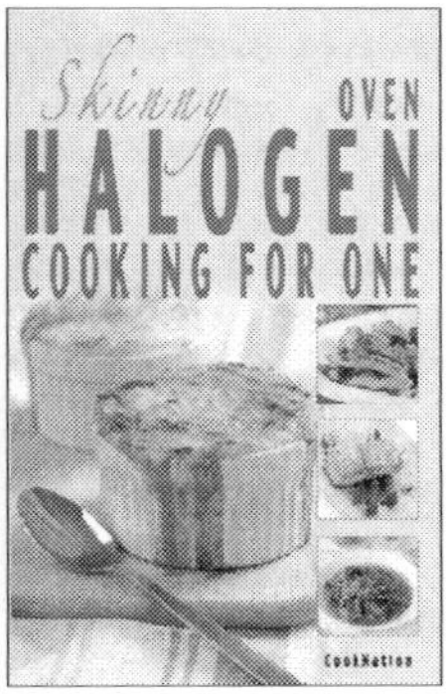

SKINNY HALOGEN OVEN COOKING FOR ONE

Single Serving, Healthy, Low Calorie Halogen Oven RecipesUnder 200, 300 and 400 Calories.

Paperback / eBook

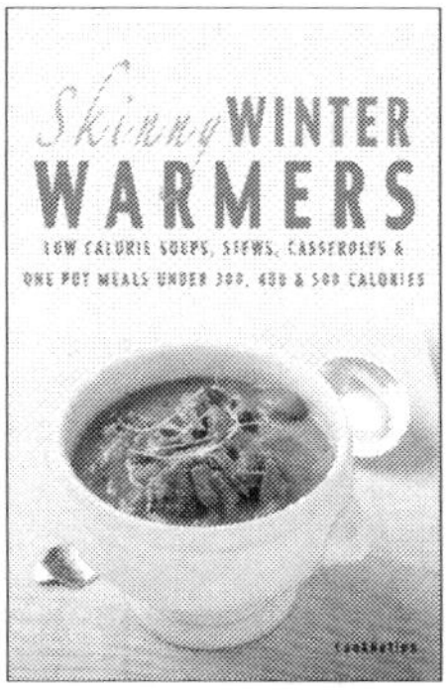

SKINNY WINTER WARMERS RECIPE BOOK

Soups, Stews, Casseroles & One Pot Meals Under 300, 400 & 500 Calories.

Paperback / eBook

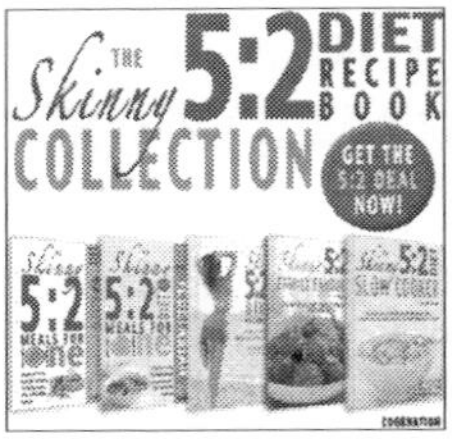

THE SKINNY 5:2 DIET RECIPE BOOK COLLECTION

All The 5:2 Fast Diet Recipes You'll Ever Need. All Under 100, 200, 300, 400 And 500 Calories.

eBook

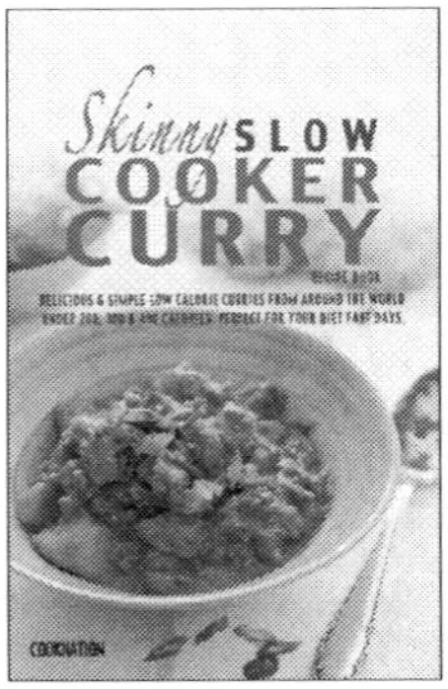

THE SKINNY SLOW COOKER CURRY RECIPE BOOK

Low Calorie Curries From Around The World.

Paperback / eBook

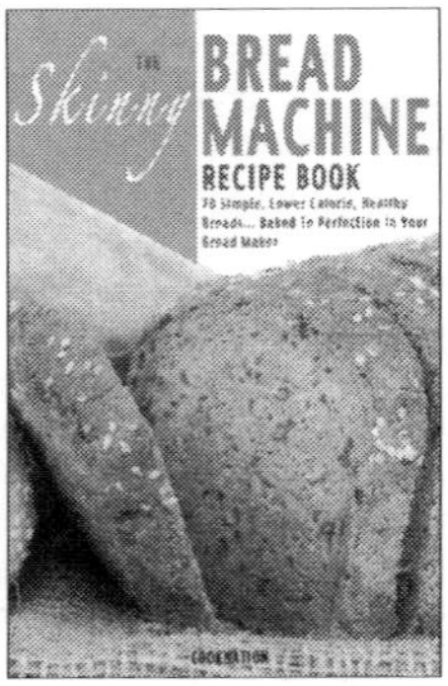

THE SKINNY BREAD MACHINE RECIPE BOOK

70 Simple, Lower Calorie, Healthy Breads...Baked To Perfection In Your Bread Maker.

Paperback / eBook

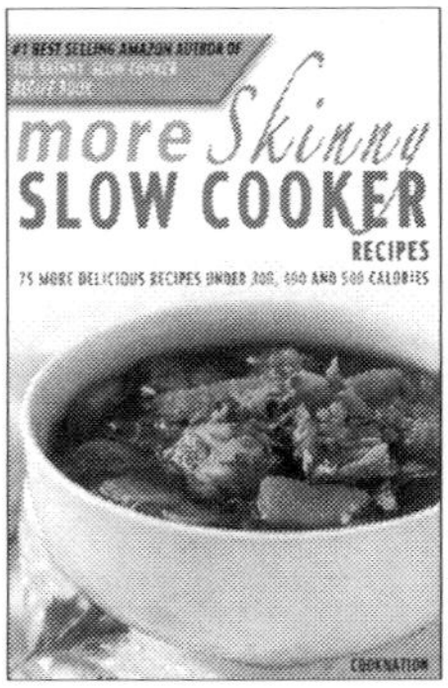

MORE SKINNY SLOW COOKER RECIPES

75 More Delicious Recipes Under 300, 400 & 500 Calories.

Paperback / eBook

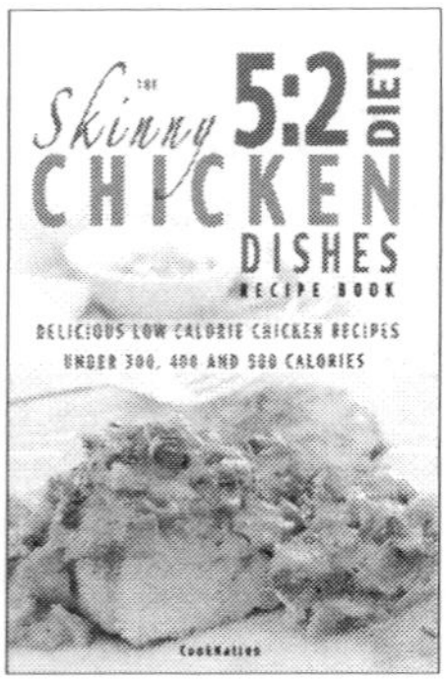

THE SKINNY 5:2 DIET CHICKEN DISHES RECIPE BOOK

Delicious Low Calorie Chicken Dishes Under 300, 400 & 500 Calories.

Paperback / eBook

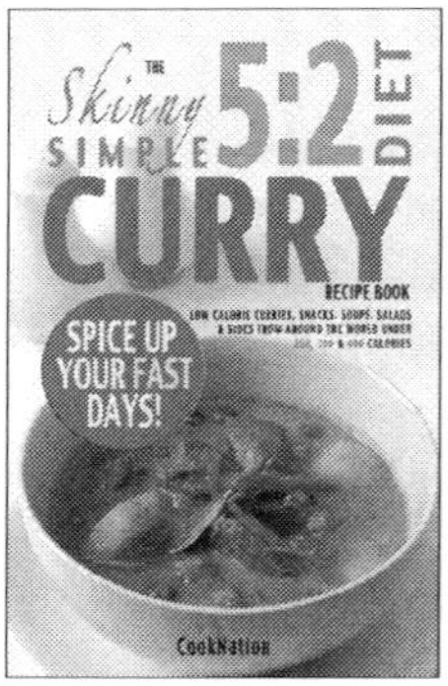

THE SKINNY 5:2 CURRY RECIPE BOOK

Spice Up Your Fast Days With Simple Low Calorie Curries, Snacks, Soups, Salads & Sides Under 200, 300 & 400 Calories.

Paperback / eBook

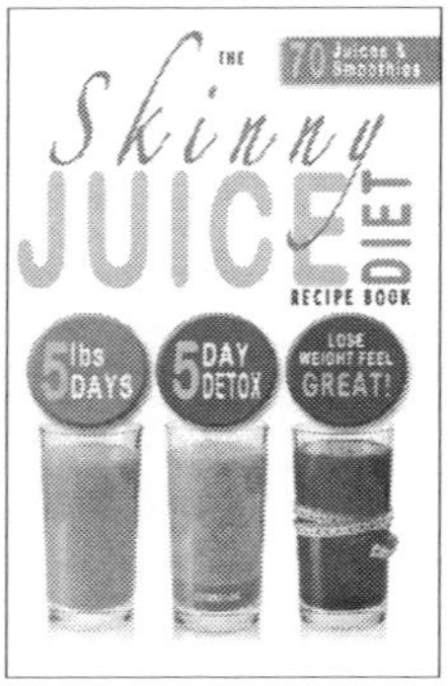

THE SKINNY JUICE DIET RECIPE BOOK

5lbs, 5 Days. The Ultimate Kick- Start Diet and Detox Plan to Lose Weight & Feel Great!

Paperback / eBook

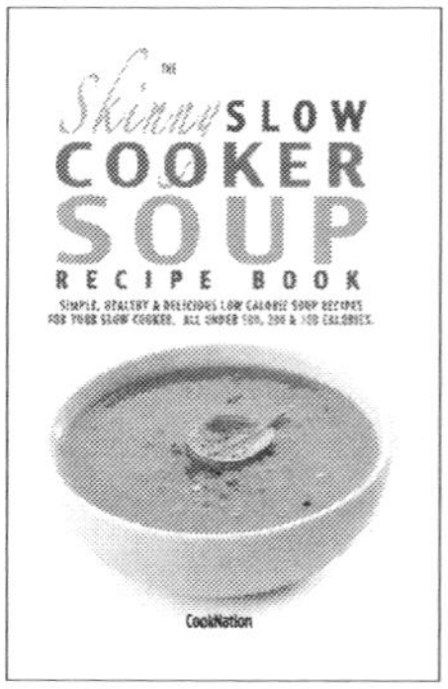

THE SKINNY SLOW COOKER SOUP RECIPE BOOK

Simple, Healthy & Delicious Low Calorie Soup Recipes For Your Slow Cooker. All Under 100, 200 & 300 Calories.

Paperback / eBook

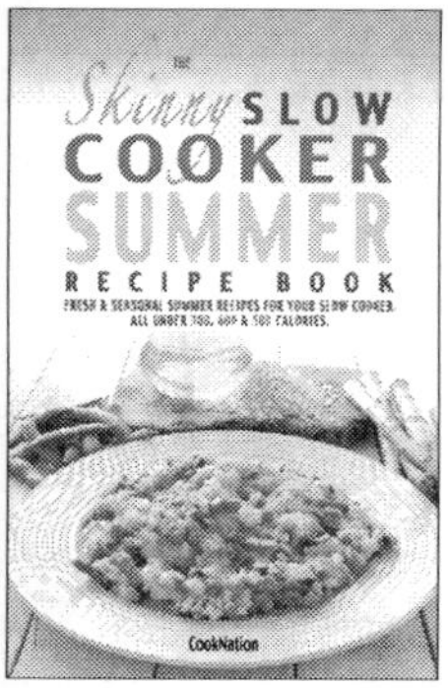

THE SKINNY SLOW COOKER SUMMER RECIPE BOOK

Fresh & Seasonal Summer Recipes For Your Slow Cooker. All Under 300, 400 And 500 Calories.

Paperback / eBook

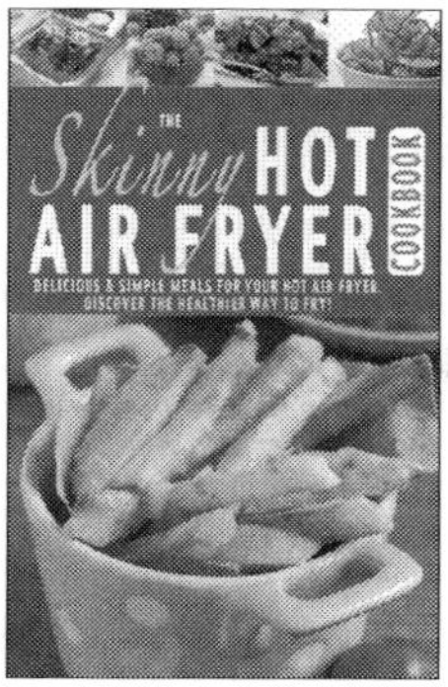

THE SKINNY HOT AIR FRYER COOKBOOK

Delicious & Simple Meals For Your Hot Air Fryer: Discover The Healthier Way To Fry.

Paperback / eBook

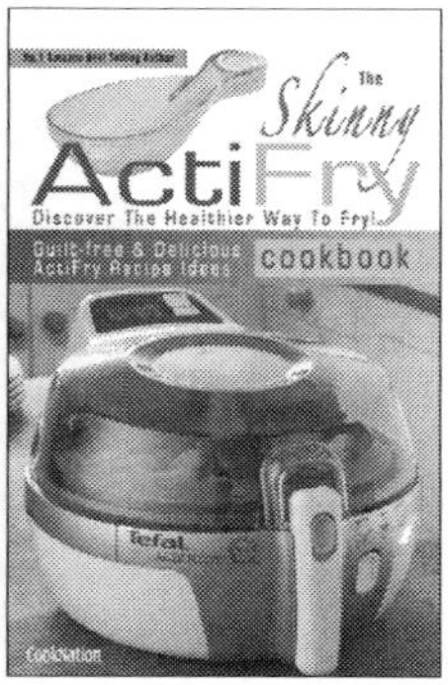

THE SKINNY ACTIFRY COOKBOOK

Guilt-free and Delicious ActiFry Recipe Ideas: Discover The Healthier Way to Fry!

Paperback / eBook

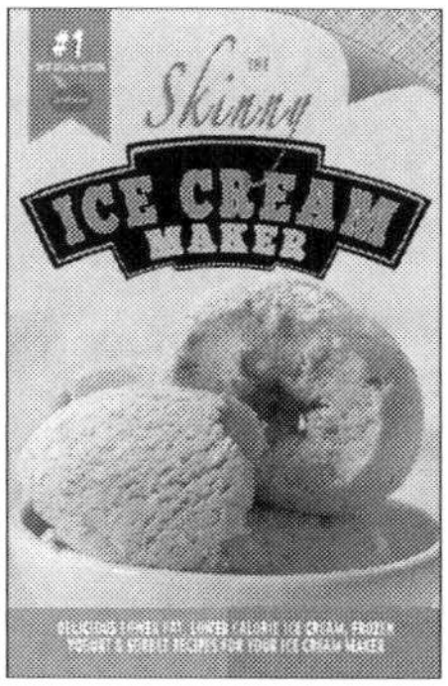

THE SKINNY ICE CREAM MAKER

Delicious Lower Fat, Lower Calorie Ice Cream, Frozen Yogurt & Sorbet Recipes For Your Ice Cream Maker.

Paperback / eBook

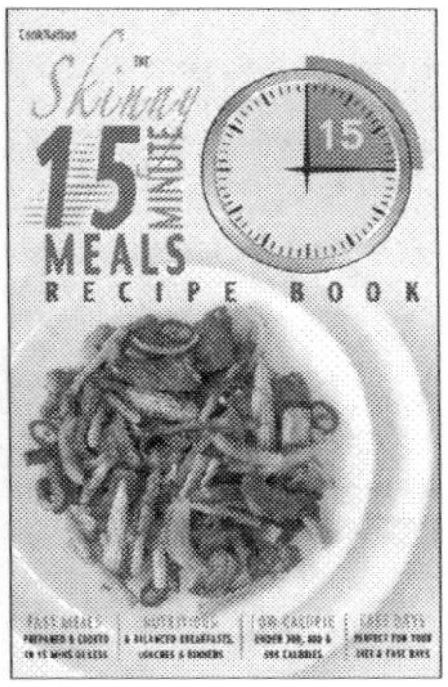

THE SKINNY 15 MINUTE MEALS RECIPE BOOK

Delicious, Nutritious & Super-Fast Meals in 15 Minutes Or Less. All Under 300, 400 & 500 Calories.

Paperback / eBook

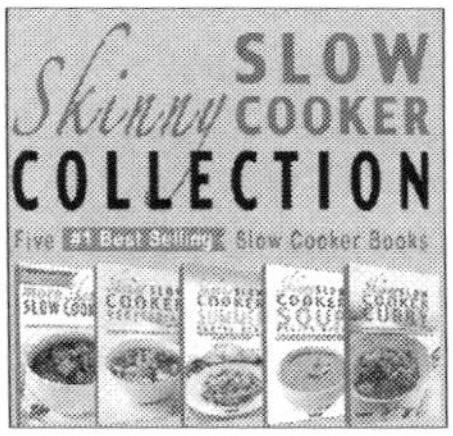

THE SKINNY SLOW COOKER COLLECTION

5 Fantastic Books of Delicious, Diet-friendly Skinny Slow Cooker Recipes: ALL Under 200, 300, 400 & 500 Calories!

eBook

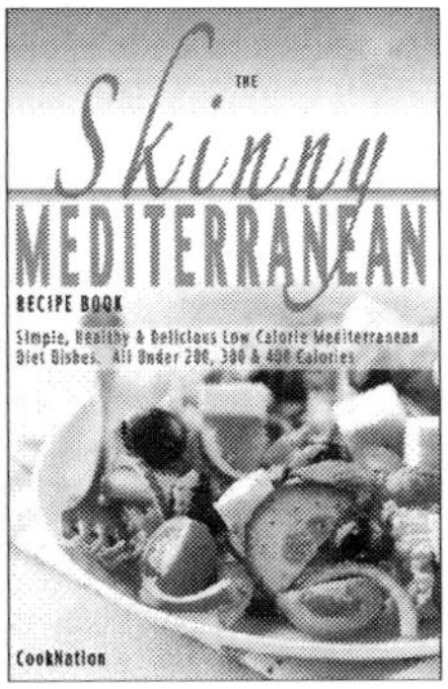

THE SKINNY MEDITERRANEAN RECIPE BOOK

Simple, Healthy & Delicious Low Calorie Mediterranean Diet Dishes. All Under 200, 300 & 400 Calories.

Paperback / eBook

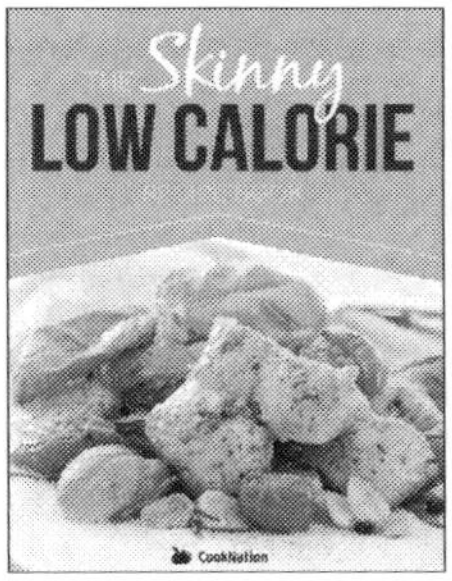

THE SKINNY LOW CALORIE RECIPE BOOK

Great Tasting, Simple & Healthy Meals Under 300, 400 & 500 Calories. Perfect For Any Calorie Controlled Diet.

Paperback / eBook

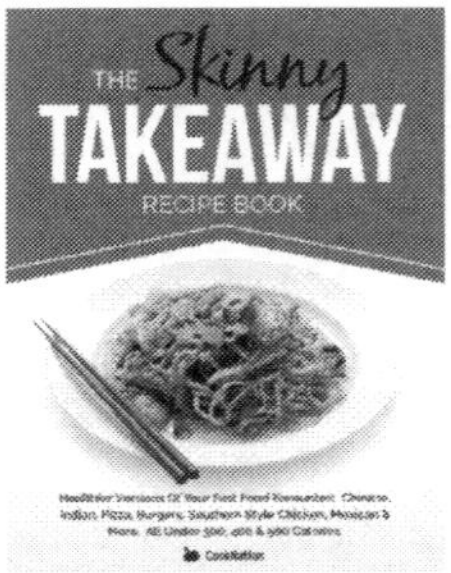

THE SKINNY TAKEAWAY RECIPE BOOK

Healthier Versions Of Your Fast Food Favourites: All Under 300, 400 & 500 Calories.

Paperback / eBook

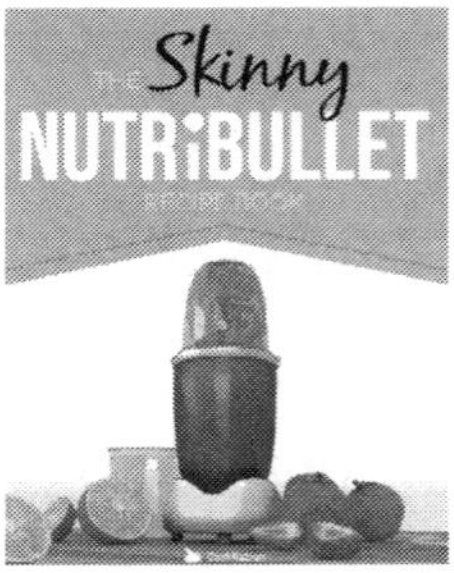

THE SKINNY NUTRIBULLET RECIPE BOOK

80+ Delicious & Nutritious Healthy Smoothie Recipes. Burn Fat, Lose Weight and Feel Great!

Paperback / eBook

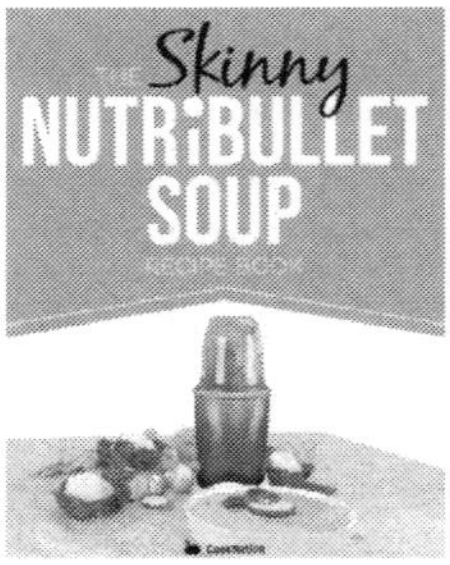

THE SKINNY NUTRIBULLET SOUP RECIPE BOOK

Delicious, Quick & Easy, Single Serving Soups & Pasta Sauces For Your Nutribullet. All Under 100, 200, 300 & 400 Calories!

Paperback / eBook

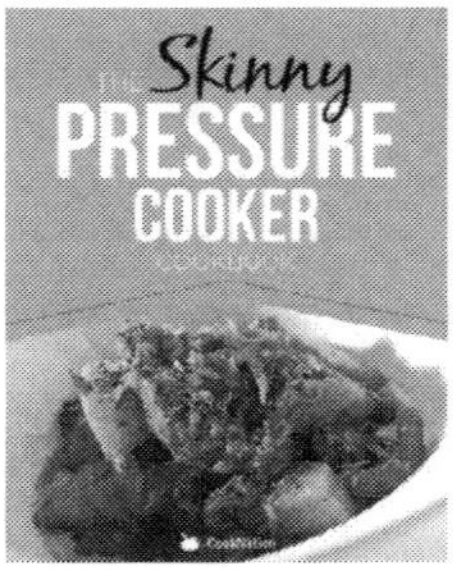

THE SKINNY PRESSURE COOKER COOKBOOK

USA ONLY

Low Calorie, Healthy & Delicious Meals, Sides & Desserts. All Under 300, 400 & 500 Calories.

Paperback / eBook

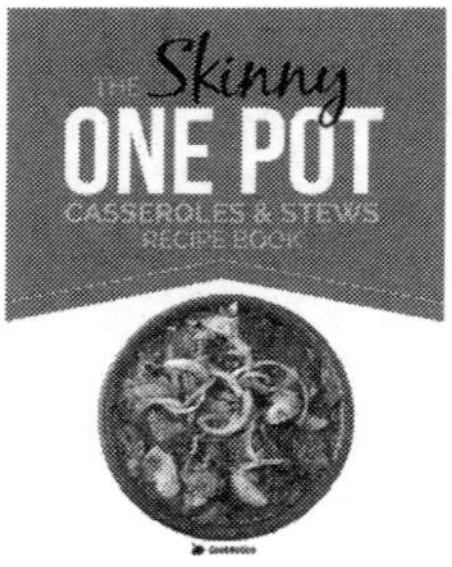

THE SKINNY ONE-POT RECIPE BOOK

Simple & Delicious, One-Pot Meals. All Under 300, 400 & 500 Calories

Paperback / eBook

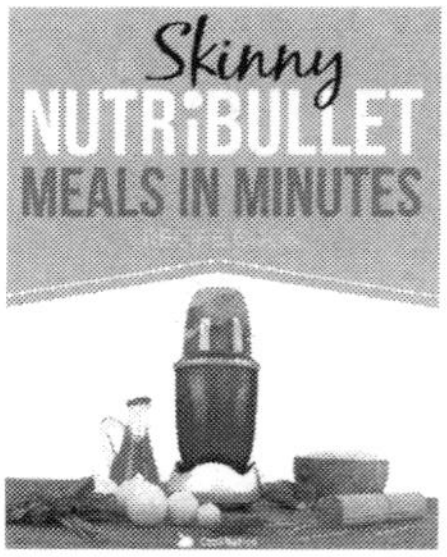

THE SKINNY NUTRIBULLET MEALS IN MINUTES RECIPE BOOK

Quick & Easy, Single Serving Suppers, Snacks, Sauces, Salad Dressings & More Using Your Nutribullet. All Under 300, 400 & 500 Calories

Paperback / eBook

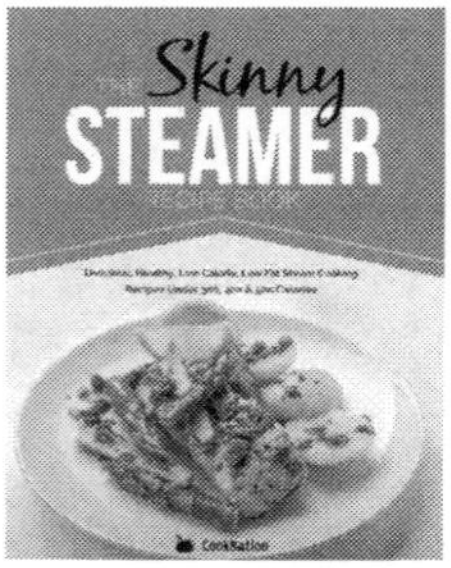

THE SKINNY STEAMER RECIPE BOOK

Healthy, Low Calorie, Low Fat Steam Cooking Recipes Under 300, 400 & 500 Calories.

Paperback / eBook

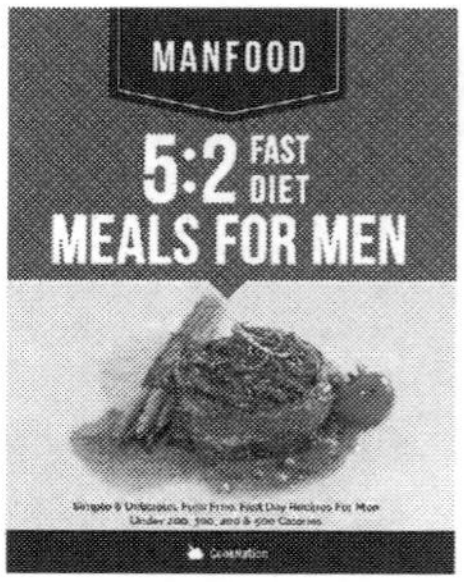

MANFOOD: 5:2 FAST DIET MEALS FOR MEN

Simple & Delicious, Fuss Free, Fast Day Recipes For Men Under 200, 300, 400 & 500 Calories.

Paperback / eBook

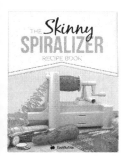

THE SKINNY SPIRALIZER RECIPE BOOK

Delicious Spiralizer Inspired Low Calorie Recipes For One. All Under 200, 300, 400 & 500 Calories

Paperback / eBook

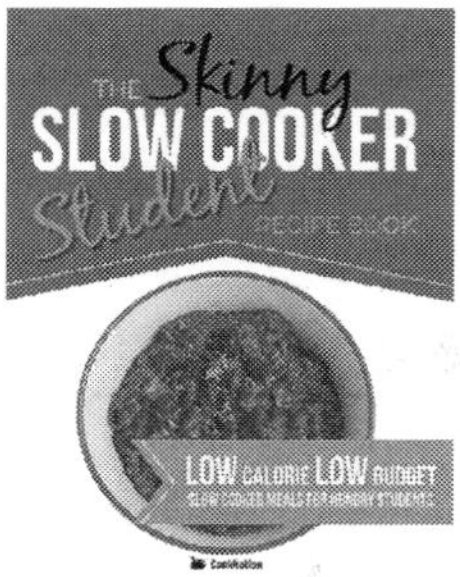

THE SKINNY SLOW COOKER STUDENT RECIPE BOOK

Delicious, Simple, Low Calorie, Low Budget, Slow Cooker Meals For Hungry Students. All Under 300, 400 & 500 Calories

Paperback / eBook

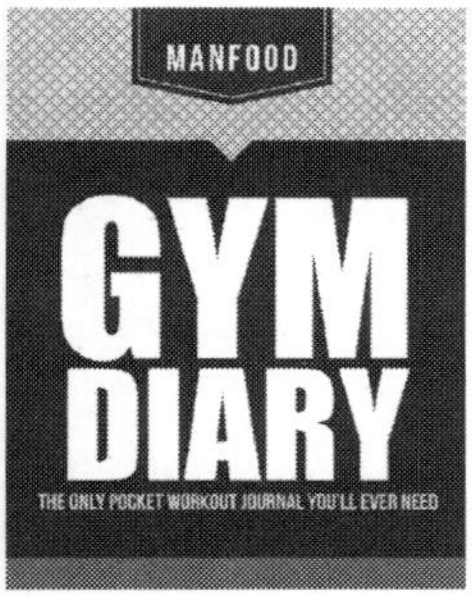

MANFOOD: GYM DIARY:

The Only Pocket Workout Journal You'll Ever Need

Paperback / eBook

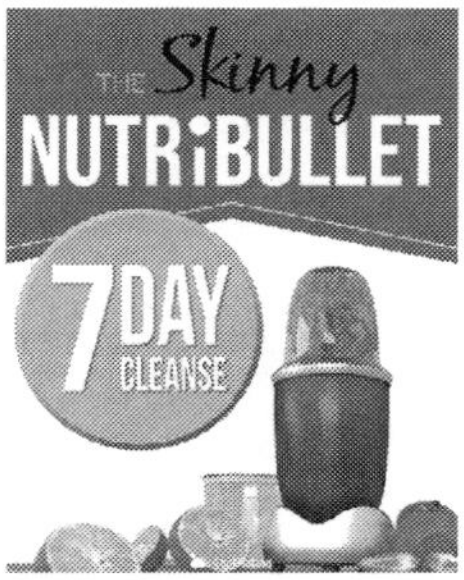

THE SKINNY NUTRIBULLET 7 DAY CLEANSE

Calorie Counted Cleanse & Detox Plan: Smoothies, Soups & Meals to Lose Weight & Feel Great Fast. Real Food. Real Results

Paperback / eBook

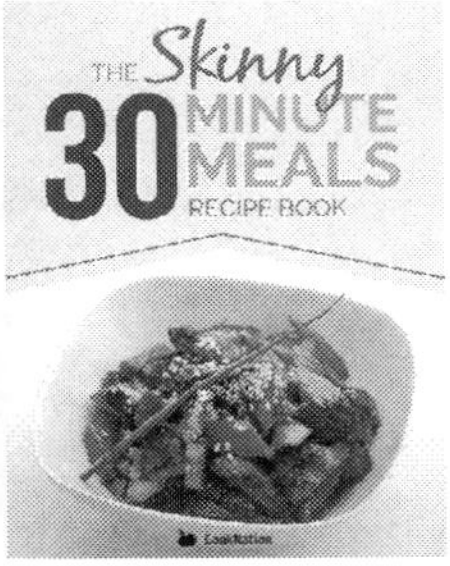

THE SKINNY 30 MINUTE MEALS RECIPE BOOK

Great Food, Easy Recipes, Prepared & Cooked In 30 Minutes Or Less. All Under 300, 400 & 500 Calories

Paperback / eBook

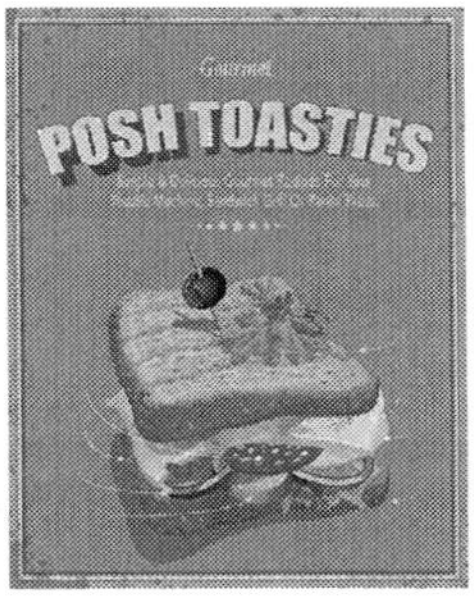

POSH TOASTIES

Simple & Delicious Gourmet Recipes For Your Toastie Machine, Sandwich Grill Or Panini Press

Paperback / eBook

Printed in Great Britain
by Amazon

28259342R00055